The **Father's** Home Birth Handbook

Leah Hazard

The **Father's** Home Birth Handbook

Published in 2008 by
Victoria Park Press
51 Victoria Park Drive North
Glasgow G14 9NW
www.homebirthbook.com

The author has made every effort to ensure the accuracy of the information presented in this book. However, the author cannot accept responsibility for any accident, injury or loss resulting from the use of this book. Medical advice and personal judgment should be considered when making any decisions about care during the childbearing year.

ISBN 978-0-9560711-0-1

British Library Cataloguing-in-Publication Data
A catalogue record for this book is available from the British Library

Typeset, printed and bound in Great Britain by Biddles, King's Lynn, Norfolk

Design by Susan Roan
Cover photograph by Cara Connolly

Contents

Acknowledgments

I would like to thank the staff of Glasgow City Council libraries for providing me with a variety of lovely workspaces in which to write this book.

Many thanks go to Nadine Edwards for her wisdom and expertise; to Adela Stockton for her invaluable role as proof-reader, mentor and friend; to Maddie McMahon for helping with everything from contributors to commas; to Emma Keogh for design wizardry; and to the Scottish Doula Network and Doula UK for their support. Thank you to Patrick Houser for his enthusiasm, and to Jan Tritten for encouraging and inspiring me.

Thank you to two wise and wonderful women, Cara Connolly and Susan Roan, for believing in this project from its earliest days, and for making the finished product look like a 'real book'. I owe you a thousand lunches.

I also owe a great debt to the parents whom I have had the privilege of supporting through pregnancy and birth over the last few years; without you, this book would not exist. And, of course, my sincerest gratitude to the fathers who have shared their stories here: your candour and sensitivity have been a delight.

Finally, thank you to my family: my in-laws, for bearing with me while I do my 'wee job'; my parents, for giving me their unflagging love and support; my brother, for sharing his friendship and his publishing know-how; and my beautiful daughters, Anna and Sasha, for changing my life for the better in a million ways. And thanks to my husband, Alan, for catching the baby – and for everything else.

Prologue

When I first had the idea for this book, I joked to my friends that the title would be, *She wants to do WHAT?!: a home birth guide for fathers.* In the course of my work supporting pregnant women and their partners through the childbearing year, I've met a handful of men who have been enthusiastic about the potential benefits and joys of home birth. However, I've met far more men who have responded to their partners' home birth wishes with a mixture of shock, cynicism and fear. On the face of it, these men have been kind, supportive and intelligent, with a genuine concern for the wellbeing of their partners and babies. They have expressed willingness to rub backs for hours on end, to do battle with scalpel-happy obstetricians and to tolerate labour-induced obscenities with a calm smile but, somehow, the idea of birthing at home has been a step too far for these fathers-to-be. Why?

Far from being domineering ogres who just want to see wifey tucked 'safely' away in a hospital, these loving fathers have simply had very little access to accurate, impartial information about the safety and logistics of home births versus hospital births. What's more, whereas women often hear stories from female friends and relatives who have given birth in a variety of locations and situations, men are a bit less likely to sit down in the office/bar/clubhouse to swap birth stories. What they know, by and large, is a composite of brief snippets gleaned from the media and wry comments from friends who've already 'taken the plunge'. Men worry about what their co-workers will think if they 'let' their partner have a home birth, they worry about the hassle they'll get from their well-meaning mothers (most of whom gave birth in the medically interventionist heyday of the 1960s and 1970s) and they worry about the smell, the mess and the sheer emotional and physical intensity of birth at home. Perhaps more than anything, they worry about the safety of birth without the tricks and tools of modern technology. Fathers' fears and concerns have received scant attention from the mainstream media but, at a time when our hospital-based maternity services are in crisis, men need to be informed and encouraged if home birth is ever to be a real option for women.

The aim of this book is not to harangue you into supporting home birth. Admittedly, birthing at home will never appeal to all of the people, all of the time, nor is it clinically advisable under certain circumstances. Different countries will also have their own regulations and recommendations with respect to home birth. However, I believe that the freedom to choose your child's place of birth is a universal human right that transcends political and medical trends. If you and your partner do choose to meet your baby in your own home, then this book will, I hope, provide you with some of the tools that you'll need to make that happen, wherever in the world you may be.

But don't take it from me. I'm just one person with her own inevitable biases and back-story, and – as you may have guessed from my name – I am not a father. In addition to presenting some information that you might find useful as you make your birth choices, I shall also have the pleasure of introducing you to the 28 fathers who have been kind enough to contribute their stories to this book. These home-birthing dads range in age from 23 to 53; they hail from the UK, the US, Canada, New Zealand, Finland and the Netherlands; and they include an artist, a banker, a gardener, a US Marine and a cardiac physiologist. The birth stories you'll read in this book are as diverse as the fathers who've shared them, from 'blink-and-you've-missed-it' births to marathon three-day labours, from straightforward deliveries to complicated dramas. You will hear these fathers' voices throughout this book: whether joyous, terrified, sceptical or enthusiastic, each one is a true reflection of the home birth experience.

One of these voices will be that of Alan – my husband – who caught our second baby himself when the midwife didn't quite make it to the house in time. A mechanic by trade, Alan now swears that this experience taught him that birth is 'the greatest single feat of engineering in the world'. Will you agree? The day may soon come when you'll find out for yourself. In the meantime, allow me to share some facts, offer some insights, and introduce you to a few more fathers who've come to the idea of home birth with open minds and loving hearts.

1

Risk and Responsibility

Let's get right down to it: the question on almost everyone's lips when they first think of home birth is, 'Is it safe?' Perhaps you're just beginning to turn that question over in your own mind, or perhaps you've already encountered shocked expressions and tales of doom from well-meaning friends, relations and colleagues. But, no matter whether you think birth is a natural joy or you think that the Caesarean section is God's gift to women, you will need to satisfy yourself that your choice is the safest one possible.

Before we can even begin to address the question of safety, we first need to answer the even thornier question of what safety actually is. You might expect an official body, such as the UK's Department of Health, to come up with a black-and-white definition of the term, but even its position allows for a huge grey area: 'Safety is not an absolute concept. It is part of a greater picture encompassing all aspects of health and wellbeing.'[1] Does safety simply equal a live mother and a live baby, at all costs? Is a safe birth one from which all parties emerge physically and emotionally unscathed, or is it an experience that leaves the new family feeling physically stronger and emotionally triumphant? Is safety a matter of ticking boxes, or looking at the big picture? You and your partner will need to explore and define your own ideas of safety before you can begin to make an informal 'risk assessment' of your chosen mode of birth. What do you even consider to be a risk, and what risks are you willing to take? What does the idea of home birth mean for the physical and emotional integrity of your growing family? Finally, what do your ideas about home birth say about you – is home birth a challenge to your own identity as a man, a father and a member of the community?

Is home birth safe for mothers and babies?

Because it's easier to quantify live mothers and babies than it is to quantify happy families, let's start with the former. Can maternal and neonatal mortality rates for home births possibly begin to approach those of hospital births? After all, don't hospitals hold out the promise of highly-trained staff bustling purposefully along gleaming corridors, with up-to-the-minute technology bleeping reassuringly in the background? Can you possibly hope to achieve the same results in your own home, where the whiff of last night's curry lingers over strategically placed piles of dirty laundry? You're not alone in your concerns, as one of the fathers interviewed for this book noted:

> ***On one hand, as educated people, we know that women didn't really have babies in hospitals 80 years ago, and everyone was born at home; hospital birth is nothing but a recent aberration from a historical point of view. But, of course, we also know that death rates of women and children went down dramatically with the introduction of hospitals, so you may think, 'Maybe it's not just a matter of clean hands, maybe hospitals really do help in crucial cases,' and you never know if you're going to be one of those cases. (George)***

The only way to answer the question of whether hospital births really do produce more live mothers and babies is to look at the many studies that have been done on exactly that issue. Overwhelmingly, the results of these studies – conducted by a diverse range of individuals and organisations in a number of different countries over the last three decades – suggest that, for the majority of women with normal pregnancies, home birth is at least as safe, if not safer, than birth in a hospital. Here is a chronological list of a few of the more prominent studies that have compared mortality rates for home births and hospital births:

1986 Marjorie Tew publishes a groundbreaking article in the British Journal of Obstetrics and Gynaecology, analysing 'official statistics, national surveys, and specific studies'. Tew finds that 'perinatal mortality is much higher, when obstetric intranatal interventions are used, as in consultant hospitals, than when they are little used, as in unattached general practitioner maternity units and at home.' Tew also concludes that the decline in perinatal mortality over the previous 50 years owes more to the general improvement in mothers' health than it does to the increased use of hospital-based interventions.[2]

1996 The Northern Region Perinatal Mortality Survey (UK) publishes the results of its study, looking at 558,691 births from 1981 to 1994. The researchers found that perinatal mortality for planned home births was less than half the average for all births, and even those few deaths among the home birth group were 'mostly unavoidable'.[3]

1996 Similar perinatal mortality rates for home births and hospital births are found by a Swiss team looking at a total of 874 women in Zurich. The researchers note that 'the home birth group needed significantly less medication and fewer interventions,' and those babies born at home had slightly higher Apgar scores* than their hospital-born counterparts.[4]

1996 A study of 1,836 women with low-risk pregnancies in the Netherlands found that place of birth did not influence perinatal outcome, except in multiparous women (women who had already had one baby), where the perinatal outcome was significantly better for those giving birth at home.[5]

* An Apgar score is one way of measuring a baby's wellbeing at birth.

1997 A researcher from the University of Copenhagen publishes a meta-analysis of six studies comparing home birth and hospital birth. Among the 24,092 women participating in these studies, 'perinatal mortality was not significantly different in the two groups [women delivering at home versus women delivering in hospital],' and no maternal deaths occurred in either group. If anything, babies in the home birth group were less likely to have low Apgar scores, and the mothers were more likely to deliver without medical interventions (induction, episiotomy, Caesarean section, etc.).[6]

1999 The National Birthday Trust (UK) publishes the results of its confidential survey of 4,500 home births in the UK, concluding that 'a woman who is appropriately selected and screened for a home birth is putting herself and her baby at no greater risk than a mother of similar low-risk profile who is hospital booked and delivered.'[7]

2000 Gavin Young, a general practitioner, and Edmund Hey, part of the Regional Perinatal Mortality Survey Coordinating Group (UK), note, 'There has been no intrapartum death and only one neonatal (0-27 day) death in the past 15 years among the estimated 3,400 mothers . . . who were booked for home birth when labour started.'[8]

2005 British Medical Journal publishes the largest ever study of planned home births attended by a certified professional midwife (CPM). Looking at the results from all 5,418 women expecting to deliver at home with a CPM in the United States and Canada in the year 2000, the researchers find that 'planned home birth for low-risk women in North America using certified professional midwives was associated with lower rates of medical intervention but similar intrapartum and neonatal mortality to that of low-risk hospital births in the United States.'[9]

Evidence from these studies points clearly to the fact that home birth is safe for healthy women and healthy babies around the world. Although hospital birth may still be the norm for most women, the consensus in favour of home birth is increasingly echoed by the policies of professional organisations. Case in point:

> ***The Royal College of Midwives (RCM) and the Royal College of Obstetricians and Gynaecologists (RCOG) support home birth for women with uncomplicated pregnancies. There is no reason why home birth should not be offered to women at low risk of complications and it may confer considerable benefits for them and their families. There is ample evidence showing that labouring at home increases a woman's likelihood of a birth that is both satisfying and safe, with implications for her health and that of her baby.***[10]

The British government began to accept a woman's right to choose a home birth several years ago, conceding that 'all women should be involved in planning their own care with information, advice and support from professionals, including choosing the place they would like to give birth,'[11] and the Department of Health went one step further in its Maternity Matters paper (2007), suggesting that 'birth supported by a midwife at home' should be 'one of the key national choice guarantees' in place by 2009.[12]

Given these positive endorsements, prospective parents might think that the way is paved for a new 'Age of Home Birth', with doctors, midwives and politicians offering handshakes and congratulations to every woman who chooses to have her baby at home. However, in spite of the apparently overwhelming evidence to the contrary, there are still many naysayers who view home birth as a disaster waiting to happen. The American College of Obstetricians and Gynecologists recently raised the anti-home birth banner with the following statement:

The American College of Obstetricians and Gynecologists (ACOG) reiterates its long-standing opposition to home births. While childbirth is a normal physiologic process that most women experience without problems, monitoring of both the woman and the fetus during labor and delivery in a hospital or accredited birthing center is essential because complications can arise with little or no warning, even among women with low-risk pregnancies.[13]

ACOG even went as far as to propose legislation which, if passed, would officially mandate that 'the safest setting for labour, delivery and the immediate post-partum period is in the hospital, or a birthing centre within a hospital complex.' Spokesman Gregory Phillips later summarised the organisation's sentiments by saying, 'We are against home births, period.'[14]

Does ACOG know something you don't know? Is high-tech monitoring really essential for a safe birth (if, by 'safe', we are still sticking to the basic criteria of a live mother and a live baby)? Contrary to what you might expect from a leading medical body, in what is arguably one of the most medically advanced countries in the world, the folks at ACOG haven't done their homework. *A Guide to Effective Care in Pregnancy and Childbirth,* one of the most comprehensive reviews to date of clinical research, states:

In the majority of pregnancies, intrapartum death is prevented equally effectively by intermittent auscultation and by continuous electronic fetal heart-rate monitoring . . . Continuous electronic monitoring results in an increase in Caesarean section rates and postpartum morbidity for the mother, with no compensating benefits to the baby except a decreased incidence of neonatal seizures.[15]

In other words, use of the continuous electronic fetal heart monitor (notoriously lampooned by Monty Python as 'the machine that goes ping') is no more valuable than the 'old-fashioned' method of listening in at regular intervals with a hand-held device. ACOG appears to have overlooked this little piece of information, but you could forgive this organisation its oversight if its members were indeed proven to be the world leaders in neonatal and maternal safety. Strike two for ACOG: among 222 countries surveyed, 42 have lower infant mortality rates than the United States. ACOG's home turf came in behind such unlikely contenders as Malta, Slovenia and Macau, and the US came 17 places behind the Netherlands, where the state-run health system actively promotes home birth as a choice for healthy women.[16] Strike three for ACOG: the American maternal mortality rate is 1 in 2,500 – higher than in 29 other similarly-developed countries. In fact, a woman in America has a 40 percent greater chance of dying in childbirth than a woman in the Netherlands,[17] where approximately 30 percent of births occur at home. Playing by the rules of their own national pastime: three strikes, and ACOG's out.

Why, then, are some obstetricians so convinced that home births are dangerous? The answer is simply that the majority of them have very few chances (if any) to witness completely normal home births during the course of their careers. By virtue of the fact that obstetricians are hospital-based, their only contact with home birth is during their treatment of women who have had to transfer into hospital after complications have already arisen at home. Marsden Wagner, former Director of Women's and Children's Health for the World Health Organisation, provides this vivid analogy:

> ***So for the obstetricians who have never attended a home birth . . . they erroneously assume these cases [of transfer] are representative of all out-of-hospital birth. This is like the auto mechanic who sees several Mercedes with mechanical problems and concludes all Mercedes are no good, forgetting that for every Mercedes he sees in his shop, there are a thousand Mercedes running fine and therefore not brought to his shop.***[18]

To extend this analogy still further, you may wish to remember that your partner is the end product of millions of years of evolution; many Mercedes have come before her, and her body has benefited from these years and years of evolutionary 'tuning'. She is perfectly designed for the task at hand: cruising down the home birth highway.

But isn't the hospital really the safest place to give birth?

Even though planned, midwife-supported home birth has been proven to be a safe choice for the majority of healthy women, many parents still struggle to get past the popular perception that hospitals are the safest places for birth. It's likely that you and most, if not all, of your friends and colleagues were born in a hospital. Whenever you have seen birth on television or in a film, chances are that the woman in question doubled over in sudden, agonising pain before making her way at lightning speed (and possibly in an ambulance) to the nearest hospital, where she was taken in hand by brisk, white-coated doctors with easy access to a dazzling array of drugs and instruments. As one father mused:

> ***I wasn't totally committed to the idea [of home birth] to start with. Our local hospital is a modern, up-to-date facility with the latest equipment with all the required beeping and buzzing and plenty of flashing lights. When you watch dramas on the television, babies are born in the hospital or in the car on the way to the hospital, never intentionally at home. (David)***

In a society where the culturally 'normal' standard of hospital birth is constantly reinforced by the media, it may be difficult to accept the idea that that the norm is not universally beneficial.

Increases in hospital-acquired infections have grabbed countless headlines over the past few years and, for many parents considering home birth, hospitals no longer hold out the promise of a clean, sterile environment. For example, the 'clean hands' mentioned earlier by Leon as a perk of hospital birth may now be lost in the mists of time, a fact made even more alarming when we consider the number of clinicians who might touch, examine or operate on a woman during the course of an average hospital birth. When researchers at the University of Florida swabbed the gloves of obstetricians prior to Caesarean deliveries, they found that 36% of these gloves tested positive for staphylococcal bacteria (the family to which the famously drug-resistant MRSA bug belongs).[19] Another study of 540 sets of gloves used during obstetric surgical procedures found that approximately 12% of the procedures were performed with perforated gloves; moreover, only 3% of glove tears were actually recognised by the surgeon.[20] A woman undergoing a typical hospital birth is not only at risk of infection from damaged or contaminated gloves; it is also likely that she will be treated with a medical device such as an intravenous cannula (for the administration of fluids, synthetic hormone drips, etc.) or a urinary catheter. While these devices may be used ostensibly to 'help' the woman in question, it's worth bearing in mind the results of a study of three million patients in English hospitals from 1997 to 2002: almost two-thirds of bacterial infections detected were 'associated with an intravascular device or with device-related infections'. Unfortunately, the babies in the study didn't fare much better; neonatal intensive care units were found to be one of the areas with the highest risk of infection.[21] News from across the Pond isn't much better; a study released in 2007 found that 34 of every 1,000 American hospital patients are infected with MRSA.[22] Hand-washing becomes a moot point when even the surgeon's rubber gloves are contaminated, and the previously reassuring infrastructure of needles and tubes now appears to be a potential bacterial swamp. A woman who comes into the hospital to have her baby may walk away with more than a bundle of joy; surgical devices and deliveries may leave her vulnerable to infection at the very time when her body is already performing one of its toughest tasks.

Anecdotal evidence supports the notion that hospitals are no longer the bastions of cleanliness and hygiene that they were once thought to be.

Murray from Scotland was disturbed by the cleanliness of the hospital where his wife received her antenatal care:

> ***When we went in, the place wasn't set up well. It's an old hospital, and from my experiences in my profession [as a cardiac physiologist], I could see that the rooms weren't set up properly. There were tiles falling off the wall, and you know you can't clean properly if there are tiles falling off the wall. You've got MRSA and all the things have to be wipeable. I know the new guidelines and these rooms didn't fit the guidelines.***

Other parents have echoed Murray's concern; in fact, a father from New Zealand said that one of the most alarming things about his wife's antenatal care was 'a pamphlet from the local hospital that told us to bring our own cleaning gear. What the hell is up with that!!!' Bob, an artist from Scotland, was similarly shocked by the hospital conditions portrayed in a documentary that was televised during his wife's early pregnancy:

> ***There was a documentary on TV, Panorama, just following undercover reporters around this hospital. It showed people being left for hours and hours on end, not even in maternity suites, but basically in cupboards, and having to deliver by themselves. They never had enough equipment, and the whole thing looked absolutely terrifying. It looked quite realistic that not only would we not get what we wanted if we chose a hospital birth, but it looked like a third world operation.***

Alan from Scotland had first-hand experience of one of those 'cupboards' when he was sent to a broom closet to change into surgical scrubs prior to his wife's Caesarean section. Speaking about that traumatic birth of his first child, Alan reflected, 'You're in a hospital where you think you'll be cared for and looked after, but you're not. That was a big lesson.'

When hospitals start asking their patients to bring their own cleaning materials, when women enter hospitals healthy and leave them sick, and when cupboards begin to stand in for labour suites, then serious questions must be asked about whether the hospital is truly the place for the best possible care.

But isn't it possible to have a normal, natural birth in the hospital?

What of the woman who has a 'normal' birth in hospital, with minimal time on the ward and minimal exposure to potentially unclean devices? Rather than rushing into the labour suite at the first sign of a contraction, she labours comfortably at home, using relaxation techniques and the support of her partner to help her through the early stages. When she feels that birth is imminent, she makes her way to the hospital, where her waters break on their own, her contractions remain strong and consistent, and she continues to cope well with the pain. This woman uses gravity-efficient positions to deliver her baby without the help of surgical instruments and, after breastfeeding her new arrival, she waits for the placenta to slip away on its own. Tucked up in a bed of clean sheets with a tremendous sense of wellbeing and accomplishment, she has just enjoyed a normal, physiological birth in the hospital.

Do you know any women who could tell you such a story? They must exist, but unfortunately, they are in the significant minority. 'Hospital birth is medicalised birth,' writes Pat Thomas in her book *Your Birth Rights*. 'A woman wanting a "natural" or "normal" birth will find such a thing almost impossible to achieve in modern hospitals.'[23] The author's dim view of hospital birth is supported by research; only one in six first-time mothers in a 2001 study experienced a normal birth, with the rate rising to only one in three mothers having their second or subsequent children.[24] The image of a woman sailing through normal labour in a hospital, untouched by needle, knife or drug, has become little more than a fantasy. Of course, medical interventions can save lives and improve outcomes for mothers and babies *when necessary*, but in a world where conditions in labour wards are dictated more and more by mass protocols and less and less by individually tailored, woman-centred care, the line between necessity and convenience is blurred. English midwife Beverly Beech concludes, 'Some women and babies require help during labour. Unfortunately, procedures designed to help them have been imposed on the majority of women and babies who do not need them.'[25]

The implications for the vast number of women who experience medical interventions during labour and birth are as numerous and complex as the interventions themselves. For example, upon hearing that you and your partner are expecting a baby, a sister or female colleague may have already pulled you aside to give you the low-down on her own birth. 'I couldn't have done it without my epidural,' she may have told you, with a conspiratorial wink. 'That anaesthetist was a lifesaver.' While epidural anaesthetic can, when properly administered, provide complete pain relief, it also comes with its own laundry list of potential side effects. Because epidurals generally produce numbness from the waist down, a woman with an epidural will probably need to lie back, which reduces blood flow to the placenta and may result in fetal distress. As the woman is unable to maintain an upright position, gravity's effect on the baby's descent is greatly reduced, labour may be slowed or stalled completely, and the woman is more likely to require a hormone drip to intensify her contractions. Even after all of this 'assistance,' she may still need to have her baby pulled from her body by a forceps-wielding consultant. These procedures carry with them their own substantial risks, before one even begins to explore the many other potential side effects of the epidural, which include incomplete pain relief, fever, low blood pressure, infection from the needle site, headache, backache, and bladder dysfunction. While this example is not intended to portray epidurals as the root of all obstetric evil, it is clear that a seemingly innocuous intervention can have consequences that range from the irritating to the debilitating – even if your sister *did* fall in love with her anaesthetist.

My partner says she just feels safer at home. Does that matter? Does *feeling* safer equate to *being* safer?

Having looked at the evidence, you may feel that a hospital is still the best place for the birth of your baby. Why is your partner so 'hung up' on the idea of a home birth? You've got a decent chance of ending up with a live mother and a live baby no matter where you deliver, so what's the point in leaping into the unknown and having this baby at home? In order to answer that question, we need to look at the way that our industrialised western culture perceives birth. While indigenous cultures tend to value and celebrate birth as a physically, emotionally and spiritually transformational event in a woman's life, here in the modern West we tend to see birth as a temporary discomfort – an ordeal best endured and forgotten. 'Let's get it over with,' you may think. 'Either way, we'll have a baby at the end of it.'

Daunting and dangerous as birth may seem, the truth is that it matters to women. It matters a lot, whether they live in a mud hut or a penthouse apartment, whether they spend their days grinding corn or trading stocks and bonds. Birth is an event that can define the way a woman feels about herself. It can transform her identity as a mother, a lover and a member of the community. It is not surprising that the location of a birth should, at some level, influence the way the mother experiences this event. In her book *Birthing Autonomy,* Nadine Pilley Edwards looks at the factors associated with women's decisions to give birth at home:

> ***For women, home birth was about protection and reclaiming connections. Protecting the integrity of the woman and her relationship with her baby within the family. Protecting her autonomy and self esteem. Connecting to her baby, her body, her spirituality and sexuality, and integrating the baby into the family. Home was a metaphor for control and connection and hospital a metaphor for loss of control and separation.***[26]

Just as you have developed your own perception of birth from people and images around you, so your partner's perception of birth has been formed by the specific messages that she has absorbed from her own mother; from friends, family and colleagues; and from the media; as well as from her personal experiences. A woman's feelings about home birth are not just a bundle of emotional whims or 'hang ups'; they are the products of a lifetime of conscious and unconscious reflection.

For many women, the choice of where to have a baby comes down to gut instinct. Putting clinical studies and statistics to one side for a moment, let us investigate this slightly more ambiguous side of the 'safety' question. Perhaps your own partner has said, 'I just have this thing about hospitals,' or 'I just think I'd feel better in my own home.' If a woman *feels* safer at home, does it mean that she actually *is* safer? It's understandable to wonder why your partner's feelings about birth really matter when the end result appears to be the same regardless of where the event takes place but, over the last half century, science has proven that a woman's emotional state during birth can have a substantial effect on the physiological process of birth itself. One home-birthing father describes how he came to understand this mind-body connection:

> *Jenny raised the idea of a home birth because she was terrified of going into hospital...We watched some videos of home births, and they had some doctors explaining how the muscles all need to work together in labour, and how labour can be going fine at home and sometimes when you transfer to a sterile environment you get tense and nervous, and the muscles stop working as they should. You go into a fight-or-flight response and only the essential organs are working as they should, so then you can develop complications during labour. I thought, if Jenny's terrified of going into hospital, there's a high probability this will happen to her, so we decided to give home birth a go. (John)*

This notion that fear can actually affect the physical course of labour was first explored by Grantly Dick-Read, a British obstetrician who also sustained serious injuries during the First World War. Having witnessed pain on the labour ward and experienced it first hand on the battlefield, Dick-Read identified something he later called the Fear-Tension-Pain Syndrome. He suggested that pain in an otherwise normal labour is a result of fear; this fear produces a physical response in which the blood flow to the uterus is restricted, and the uterus becomes tense; and this tension in turn produces pain. This idea was initially ridiculed by the medical profession, but it has now been embraced as a fundamental truth about women's experience of birth. In a way, Dick-Read simply provided professional validation of an intuitive wisdom that has long been held by women around the world. Anthropologist Patricia Draper recalls the following comment from a woman in the Ju/'hoan tribe of South West Africa: 'Fear is the worst enemy of childbirth. If you are afraid, the birth will be hard and painful. But if you don't fear, the birth will be untroubled.'[27]

It stands to reason, then, that if a woman is afraid of giving birth in a hospital, for whatever reason and on whatever level, her experience of actually labouring in a hospital is more likely to be fraught with tension and, therefore, with pain. As a result, medical intervention might be needed to facilitate a process which might have occurred much more efficiently in a less threatening home environment. As Mika from Finland puts it:

> ***I realised what my wife had been telling me all the time: risk factors for a birth are heavily dependent on mother's feelings... Hospitals are probably safer for women who feel that a hospital environment is safe. But for those who are not comfortable with hospitals or even afraid of them, it's probably noticeably safer to have a home birth. And my wife really didn't like hospitals...That was not easy for me to understand, because I trust medical professionals (at least most of them) and I consider hospitals safe and friendly places. But what can I do? Facts are facts. And telling my wife that***

hospitals are actually good cannot change her mind.

No matter whether you agree or disagree with your partner's conviction that home is the best place to give birth, Dick-Read's Fear-Tension-Pain Syndrome has helped many people to understand how a woman's perception of her birth environment can influence the basic mechanical elements of birth. Mika (quoted above) claims that he and other fathers will be more likely to understand the benefits of home birth if this practical argument is put forward:

> ***Using emotional reasons to argue for home birth is not really going to help me. It should be presented as a psychophysical phenomenon – how emotions affect the blood pressure and hormones and how they again affect the birth process – how there is a logical chain from accepting mother's feelings, to having a safer birth.***

Whether, like Mika, you take a logical, scientific approach to the subject of home birth, or whether you take a more emotional view, what's undeniably clear is that the two sides of the topic are intimately connected. It's virtually impossible to draw a line between *feeling* safe and *being* safe when a labouring woman's state of mind has such a clear effect on her body's performance.

Can my partner still have a home birth if she's been told she's high risk?

As you may have noticed, the studies and statistics that have been discussed thus far relate mostly to a 'low-risk' home birth population, where the women in question have had normal, healthy pregnancies. If your partner has been told she is ineligible for a home birth because she's high risk, then she's in good company: many women are told by their healthcare providers that their medical history or current medical condition precludes a home delivery. Perhaps your wife has been tarred with the 'high-risk' brush because it's her first baby; it's her fourth or subsequent baby; she's too young; she's too old; she's anaemic; she's tested positive for Group B Strep; she has an Rh-negative blood type; she has a small pelvis; she has a tilted uterus; she has gestational diabetes; she has had a previous Caesarean section; she has had a previous miscarriage; her baby is breech; her baby is overdue; her baby is small; her baby is large . . . the list goes on and on. One wonders how the human race has managed to survive and evolve for all these years if so many women and their babies have been too 'risky' for birth in its most natural environment: the home.

There are certainly some specific circumstances in which it may be inadvisable to give birth at home; for example, if the mother has placenta praevia (where the placenta lies close to the cervix, or partially or fully covers the cervix), severe pre-eclampsia (pregnancy-induced hypertension), substance-abuse issues, or extreme obesity, or when there is substantial reason to believe that the baby may need special care immediately after the birth. In these and certain other instances, the hospital's resources may be valuable in giving a mother and her child the best possible chance of a safe birth. However, in many cases, a diagnosis of 'high risk' is often made because a woman appears to fall into a statistical category, and not because the healthcare practitioner has made a full appraisal of the condition of this particular woman and/or her baby. In her book about home birth, Nicky Wesson writes, 'In many cases these objections will be related to statistical risk rather than directly to you.' She goes on to explain how the experiential wisdom of certain midwives may allow them to offer a different view of risk from that put forth by the medical majority: 'Independent midwives have a strong belief in the benefits of home births and consider that very few conditions render a woman unsuitable to have her baby at home. They find that a healthy lifestyle and an informed, positive attitude is likely to result in a successful home birth, regardless of the mother's age or her previous history.'[28]

The 'high-risk' tag can also be a self-fulfilling prophecy for many women who choose hospital birth, as they are likely to be more closely monitored and more liable to receive a range of medical interventions which, in turn, carry their own risks. Sheila Kitzinger is a writer, sociologist and birth activist who feels strongly about the dangers of a high-risk diagnosis:

> ***Attaching labels to pregnant women in this way – even when done with discretion – is damaging. A woman assigned to a high-risk category will probably have interventions that make birth more complicated, and if everyone around you expects things to go wrong, you begin to believe that they will – and they may well do so.*** [30]

You and your partner must decide whether her high-risk label is justified, and whether the possible risks of hospital-based interventions outweigh the perceived risks of a home birth. It may be worth seeking the advice of several different midwives and/or obstetricians, as well as speaking to others who have been in a similar situation, before you and your partner make your decision. In the mean time, you may be interested in the stories of a few fathers whose partners have fallen into some of the most common 'high-risk' categories:

Previous Miscarriage

Women are occasionally told that they cannot have a home birth because they have experienced one or more miscarriages, and perhaps you have your own lingering, unspoken doubts about your partner's ability to carry a pregnancy safely to full term. In most cases, however, a miscarriage is a spontaneous physiological event whose cause is unknown and unlikely to influence future pregnancies and/or births. More pertinent, perhaps, is the psychological effect that these losses have had on you and your partner. Perhaps your past experience has made you cautious, and you think that you would feel 'safer' in the hospital, with your partner under the watchful eyes of a team of midwives, nurses, and obstetricians. However, hospitals may also have a negative connotation for couples who have sought medical assistance after a miscarriage, as in the case of Chi, from England. His wife, Sophie, miscarried her first pregnancy, and her subsequent experience in the hospital had an unexpected effect on her birth choices during her next pregnancy:

> *If you think about our history of having a miscarriage the first time and actually getting to the point of having a home birth the second time around, the home birth seemed like a million miles away, totally opposite from what you might expect. We thought we would have probably gone through more the medical route, knowing the previous history.*
>
> *However, I don't like hospitals at the best of times, and for us, unfortunately, hospitals have a different connotation as well. When we found out that Sophie had a miscarriage, we got the news in almost the exact same part of the hospital as the labour ward. Deep down inside of us, we can be very practical about it and say that our decision to have a home birth has got nothing to do with that experience, but I suspect that if we went to have the baby in the hospital, it would be in the back of our minds still – this negative black thought about it.*

Regardless of where you and your partner choose to bring your new baby into the world, it is worth reflecting on any previous losses as you 'clear the way' for this new birth experience. Do you still have questions about the miscarriage(s)? Has that experience made you fearful about the upcoming birth? Would a home birth ease or exaggerate those fears? Again, your own assessment of the physical and emotional safety of home birth will help you to answer these questions.

Previous Caesarean Section

A previous Caesarean section is one of the most commonly used reasons for physicians to wave the 'high-risk' banner. Women who have had one or more Caesarean sections are often warned of the risk of full uterine rupture (where the previous scar breaks open, the mother bleeds internally, and the baby's oxygen supply is depleted, necessitating immediate delivery). Many a woman has been told that she is being irresponsible by planning a Vaginal Birth After a Caesarean (VBAC), particularly if that birth is to take place at home, and many a woman has been asked how she will feel if her baby is injured or killed as a result of this allegedly reckless decision. This tactic is nothing short of emotional blackmail; even if there were a substantial risk, nobody except the baby's parent is in a position to ask such searing questions.

Fortunately for the many women who would like to plan an HBAC (home VBAC), the risk of true uterine rupture in labour after a previous Caesarean section is slim; ranging from 0.3% to 0.7%.[30,31] It should be noted that these figures generally apply to women who had a low, transverse incision in their previous Caesarean (the 'bikini line' cut across the top of the pubic area). Women who have had a vertical incision (from navel to pubic area) and women whose incision was stitched with only a single layer of sutures, rather than the more secure and more commonly used double layer, may be at higher risk. However, once again, you and your partner must decide whether this marginal risk is one that you are willing to take. True uterine rupture can be life-threatening, but the flipside of a 0.7% chance of rupture is a 99.3% incidence of non-rupture. This is a numbers game that you and your partner may or may not wish to play.

Once again, the emotional factors associated with your partner's past experience may come to bear on her feelings about home birth. Many women who have had a Caesarean section feel deeply disappointed and even traumatised by the experience and, if your partner is one of these women, then the decision to birth at home may be about much more than location: it may be a true test of her confidence, and a turning point in her perception of herself as a mother. Several fathers who were interviewed for this book reiterated how important the home birth option became for their partners, who had felt cheated by previous surgical deliveries.

> *I think that since our first child was born by Caesarean, it was never out of Debbie's mind, just how traumatic the experience was. There wasn't a day passed where she hadn't made some reference to the way his birth was, and how very, very disappointed she was. (Willie)*

> *My partner suffered a long and painful recovery [after her Caesarean] and the feeling of disappointment that she had missed out on 'giving birth'. We felt as though our 'rite of passage' had been hijacked and my wife struggled a bit to connect with our newborn daughter. That experience strengthened my/our desire for a home birth. (Stuart)*

Reflecting on her own experience of a home water birth after not one but three previous Caesarean sections, Debbie Chippington-Derrick has written about 'the stream of people who physically interfered with [her] in the name of medicine.' She insists, 'These effects last a lifetime, they are not something that I will get over, this is something that will continue to come back to haunt me.'[32] Clearly, the scars left by Caesarean sections can run deep.

You may wonder why your partner seems preoccupied with the idea of an HBAC, but it is also worth asking what the possible effects of another medicalised hospital birth might be. As we have already seen, a woman giving birth at home is more likely to experience a normal birth, without major medical interventions. For a woman who feels that she has been failed by her body and/or by the hospital system in the past, the idea of regaining some sense of autonomy, dignity and self-worth from a home birth bears serious consideration.

Breeches and Twins

A breech birth is one in which the presenting part of the baby (the part that emerges first) is the buttocks or one or both feet, rather than the head. Many practitioners regard breech birth as especially risky because of the possibility that the baby's head will get 'stuck' after the rest of the body has been born; in fact, many midwives and obstetricians practising today have never seen a completely physiological, vaginal breech birth, as so many women are advised to go straight for the supposedly 'safer' option of an elective Caesarean. There is some debate in clinical circles as to whether Caesarean section is truly the safest mode of delivery for mother and baby, and some reports suggest that the skill of the attending midwife may be a major factor in breech birth outcomes.[33]

Mary Cronk is a Scottish midwife with a long and respected career of home births, many of them breech and/or twins. In her article 'Keep Your Hands off the Breech', she notes that breech babies can be born safely at home as long as the following conditions are satisfied: the pregnancy has reached full term, there is no incidence of placenta praevia, there are no objects in the pelvis such as fibroids or ovarian cysts, the uterus is not severely bicornuate (divided), and there are no known fetal abnormalities.[34] If you and your partner choose to have your breech baby at home, then the availability of a midwife who is confident and experienced in breech birth will be a major factor in your personal 'risk assessment'. Whereas breeches used to be fairly commonplace in the earlier twentieth century when the vast majority of births were attended by midwives at home, many midwives have now lost (or have never even had) any knowledge of techniques specific to a safe breech birth.

Likewise, if your partner is expecting twins, it will be of crucial importance to enlist the support of skilled caregivers who are comfortable with this kind of delivery. While few practitioners in the Western world might advise twin birth at home, some midwives will consider the option as long as the mother's pregnancy is healthy and straightforward, and she and her partner are aware of the potential for a more complicated delivery. There is often a chance that one or both twins may be lying breech or transverse (across the pelvis) and, in some multiple births, there is a chance that one or both babies may require resuscitation, or that the mother may experience excessive bleeding. For this reason, three midwives are normally recommended for twin births – one for the mother and one for each of her babies. Like breech birth at home, the birth of twins at home has become an unusual, but not impossible, option.

These are only a few of the many reasons why a woman might be labelled 'high risk', but no label can possibly tell the full story of a woman's pregnancy. When you and your partner are making your birth choices, you may wish to look past her label and consider the full picture of her past and present health, your baby's apparent health, the possible emotional impact of a number of different birth outcomes, and the attitude of your healthcare provider. High risk may be defined by statistics, but your partner is more than a number and, as such, her desire for a home birth is more complex than any simple calculation.

What about the father's role at a home birth? To put it bluntly, what's in it for me?

While many people think of home birth as an idea that originates with the mother and is then cautiously accepted by the father, more and more men are turning to home birth because of the benefits that it offers to them as participants in the birth experience, quite apart from any emotional or physical benefit for their partners. On a purely logistical level, some men feel that the restrictive visiting hours in hospitals are unlikely to allow them full participation in a labour that could progress through all hours of the day or night:

I wanted to be part of it and there seemed to be absolutely no provisions for the hospital to cater for me being there if it happened outside 'office hours'. I just couldn't imagine that my baby was going to behave in office hours – I've never been able to stick to them and I couldn't imagine that genetically any child of mine would either. (Bob)

In contrast to the regimented routines of a hospital birth, being at home allows a father to play a more flexible role. If labour drags on through the night, the expectant father, rather than being 'sent away' in adherence with hospital guidelines, can stay with his partner or rest nearby until the situation progresses. At home, he won't need to ask directions to the toilet or the canteen, and he won't need to leave his partner in order to feed the parking meter. As one father remarked after his wife's home birth:

I felt more comfortable to be at home. Why would I want to be in hospital? At home, I could make myself a nice cup of tea, I can sit down or do whatever. If I wanted to get out of the way, I could find a nice quiet corner. I think that helped me to be a bit more relaxed. (Chi)

Relaxation and emotional empowerment appear to play just as much a role in a father's satisfaction with the birth experience as it does in a mother's. Many of today's fathers obediently follow their partners to antenatal classes, and they are briefed in all aspects of 'labour coaching' from breathing techniques to pain relief. Society expects men to be confident and competent in their dealings with medical caregivers but, in reality, the intensity of birth can catch even the most 'prepared' father off guard. This intensity may be magnified during a hospital birth, when the father may find himself sidelined by the very caregivers he had been briefed to trust; the situation may change quickly, decisions may be made by physicians with little time for explanation or reassurance, and relaxation techniques practised diligently at home may be abandoned. Nadine Edwards writes that 'men may be equally traumatized following hospital births in which they felt unable to protect their partners,'[35] a notion that's reinforced by the following story from Hannu, a Finnish father whose first child was born in a hospital:

> ***My son was born nine years before, and my feelings about the hospital environment were negative. I felt that my wife and I were occasionally mistreated by the staff. . .Finally, when I drove home alone in the middle of the night, my son spent his first night ten floors above his mother in an oxygen-box, so instead of staying together, we all slept far away from each other. Having our son made it OK, but after this I did not consider hospitals the safest or most comfortable places any more.***

Hannu's feelings of helplessness in the hospital were echoed by other fathers. Dan from England, said, 'As a husband and provider/protector, you are in control of what happens in your own home. If something is bugging your wife, you can do something about it. In a hospital, that all goes out the window.' Tim from Northern Ireland also described the way in which being at home can facilitate the father's role as protector: 'During labour, all the theory and all the ideas that you really had completely go out the window, and you're just thinking about protecting that woman and that child. Being at home allowed that to come out. I can't see how people would find those parts of themselves in a hospital ward.' Murray from Scotland agreed: 'You're at the birth to try and help as much as possible, but [in the hospital] they're not really interested in the father at all at the birth. I think some of them would be much happier if you were not there. It's just . . . you feel like you're an accessory.'

Of course, it's possible that you may not feel comfortable being at the birth at all, no matter where it occurs. This is an entirely legitimate and understandable feeling; in fact, in many cultures, having a man present during birth would be seen as highly unusual, inappropriate, or even dangerous. The modern Western trend for encouraging men into the birth space is less than fifty years old, and it may actually go against the instincts of many fathers. As loving and 'enlightened' as these men may be, supporting their partners during labour may be a terrifying prospect, and they may feel that a home birth requires them to commit to a level of participation with which they are deeply uncomfortable. Kathleen Furin, director of Philadelphia's Center for Maternal Wellness, talks about her experiences working with reluctant labour partners:

> *Birth can be a wonderful opportunity for bonding, but it doesn't have to be a certain way. I've worked with dads who've said, I can't watch, I can't look, I just can't do it.' It doesn't mean he loves her or the child any less, it just means he can't watch. He can still be there in a supportive role, he can still share the experience, it's just going to be different from the guy who wants to be the midwife, who wants to be hands-on. As long as the couple are communicating openly about their hopes and desires, the birth will go a lot more smoothly.*[36]

Ray from America talks about his anxiety around the birth, and how the choice of home birth actually allowed him to distance himself from his wife's pain if need be:

> *I don't deal well with seeing blood, or people in extreme pain. I had tremendous reservations about being in the room during the final moments of the birth, wherever it took place. A friend of mine who had had a difficult experience with his wife's hospital delivery had clutched me on the shoulder, looked me straight in the eye, and said, 'You don't want to be in that room!' And so while I planned to be as supportive as possible during the labour, I had, with my wife's support, reserved the right to leave the room, should it become overwhelming. I not-entirely-unseriously talked about the idea of retreating to a local pub with a friend or two, to keep vigil with wireless in hand, and buy a round for the house when the good news came. Mary*

consistently got laughs when she quipped, 'I am going to have a drug-free birth, but my husband won't.'

Ray and his partner were clearly open with each other about Ray's reluctance to witness the final moments of birth, and between them, they came to a mutually satisfying agreement.

Problems arise when partners feel unable to communicate their true feelings; the father may feel obliged to stay and perform in a certain way, but his Tension may simply exacerbate the mother's own anxieties. French obstetrician Michel Odent has written extensively about the possible effects of a father's presence during labour; he notes, 'Certain men have a beneficial presence, while others only slow labor down. Sometimes an overanxious man will get worried and will then try to hide it by talking too much; his chatter can keep the woman from concentrating on her labor.'[37] Home birth may offer the best of both worlds for an anxious father and his partner; as the father is in his own environment, he can float on the periphery of the birth space without compromising his own comfort, or that of his partner. If you are one of those men for whom being present at the birth is one step too far, then it's possible that home birth will allow you to experience this transformative event on your own terms, free of the artificial constraints of hospital rules and regulations.

I understand all the research, but the bottom line is that guys like me just don't do home birth.

You've looked at the facts and figures, you've heard the arguments, and your partner has stated her case. You may accept the idea that a home birth can be safe and enjoyable, you may realise how important it is to your partner's sense of self, but there may be one final hurdle that you can't quite surmount: the notion that you're just not the kind of person who 'does' home birth. While home birth used to be the norm for nearly everyone in the industrialised modern world (and still is the norm for many women in developing countries), many 'modern' men seem to feel that home birth is the exclusive preserve of sandal-wearing, tree-hugging hippies. If you can only imagine a home birth with a bearded dad chanting mantras while his kaftan-clad wife meditates through her contractions in a haze of patchouli smoke, then you're not alone.

While the pro-home birth movement may have been championed, in part, by countercultural Earth-mother types in the 1960s and 1970s, it is wrong to assume that these are the only kind of people who have home births today. The fathers who have contributed to this book come from a remarkably diverse range of social and ethnic backgrounds; many of them never would have imagined themselves taking part in something as 'unconventional' as a home birth. One study of home births in an inner city midwifery practice echoed the idea that 'birth at home may seem to be an interest of the eccentric middle class, but our experience is that an appreciable number of working-class women will opt for home birth if the service is available.'[38] Similarly, another study by a midwifery group practice in southeast London notes, 'A third of our clients are on benefits and many more are grappling with heavy socio-economic pressures.'[39] While home births in the last half century may have originated on the hippie fringes of society, there is evidence that home birth is a popular choice for all kinds of women when offered.

While the accepted image of a home-birthing couple might be decidedly middle class and most probably white, Kathleen Furin of Philadelphia's Center for Maternal Wellness explains that home birth is also a popular choice among the centre's ethnically diverse population:

> ***Most of our diverse fathers have been on board, they really 'get it' . . . in the US as well, we have this history of institutionalised racism within the medical system, and once men connect to that and recognise that [birth choices] are***

about empowerment and respecting the woman's body, and we have this ugly history, it makes a lot of sense and they're much less likely to be resistant to home birth. . . . We talk about what are your rights, to recognise it's your baby, your body, your birth – it's a basic human right for a woman to be able to give birth in the environment she chooses, with the attendants she chooses.[40]

When birth rights are put into the larger context of human rights in this way, then home birth becomes more than just a choice of location. It becomes a statement about your right to assert your independence in the community and in society as a whole – a notion that must surely strike a chord with fathers of every ethnic and social background. The risk of stepping outside your comfort zone and challenging your identity by having a home birth is a risk that you and your partner may find surprisingly rewarding in the long run.

This chapter has explored the notion of risk and responsibility. We have questioned whether home birth can be safe for women in a variety of circumstances, and asked whether it's possible to have a definition of safety at all. You have been urged to think about what home birth means to your partner, and what it offers to you. I encourage you to use this exploration as a starting point for discussions with your partner; your birth choices will emerge from an ongoing dialogue about your fears, hopes, and expectations.

Ultimately, the question of where to give birth comes down to the issue of trust: trust in your partner and her body's ability to bear your child, trust in the birth process as a natural, normal event, and trust in yourself as a strong, supportive presence. Several of the fathers who were interviewed for this book emphasised the importance of having faith in their partners, and in a woman's ability to decide on a birth that is right for her. You may still have doubts about the safety of home birth; now may be the time to examine those doubts in the context of your relationship:

It's a perfectly natural question: 'What if something happens during a home birth?' Of course it's the man's concern because it's his child too, but it's not his question to ask. If he's asking that question, then he's suggesting that the woman hasn't asked herself that question. Of course she's asked herself that question, and if she feels that it's the right thing to do, that she's in tune with the pregnancy and what her body is saying to her, then any questions or conjecture or worries from the man's side are just neuroses. (Tim)

Being there, supporting your wife, no matter what, will get you the biggest payoff for the future. This is the most important time for your wife to know that you have her back. This is the time that you as the father can show your wife that you support her birthing choice. This is the time that can define how much you love and support your wife. (Jorge)

Not only is birth a test of your support for your partner, but it has the potential to challenge the strength of your own convictions. This challenge is laid down in no uncertain terms by Alan from Scotland:

For once in your life, believe in your own shit. You say, 'I love my wife, she's this and she's that, and she can do this and that'... Actually believe it for once, instead of just saying it. Step up to the plate and say, let's go for it. Let's do it.

2

Think Positive

Bing Crosby once sang, 'Accentuate the positive, eliminate the negative.'[1] He probably never would have imagined that his cheery advice would be passed down to twenty-first century fathers thinking about home birth, but so it is. In a culture where medicalised hospital birth is the norm, and where people seem to take great delight in sharing obstetric horror stories with their nearest and dearest, it can be difficult to feel confident about any birth, let alone one that will take place in the low-tech environment of your home. Fear abounds. When you 'go public' about your decision to have a home birth, the very people you turn to for support may well be your most outspoken critics, and the resources you turn to for information may cast further doubts on your plans. The negative impact of such words and images can hardly be understated; if you begin to feel that your home birth is a disaster waiting to happen, then your anxiety may well have a destructive effect on events when labour day arrives. If, however, you choose to surround yourself with positive people, thoughts and images, then your expectation of a healthy, joyous home birth may well become a self-fulfilling prophesy. In short, Bing had the right idea.

How can I deal with my friends and relatives who think we're mad to plan a home birth?

Perhaps your friends and relatives are like-minded souls who believe in the power and possibility of normal birth. Maybe some of them have had happy, normal births; perhaps a few of those births even took place at home. If so, congratulations! You and your partner have a ready-made cheering section for your home birth, and you will be able to rely on your loved ones' support and wisdom as you look forward to your child's safe arrival.

Unfortunately, for many home-birthing fathers, their loved ones' views on home birth range from indifference, at best, to outrage, at worst:

> ***My best friend said we were totally nuts. He said, 'What are you doing? You should be in hospital!' And in terms of hiring a doula, he was in hysterics. He thought it was ridiculous, and that we should just go into hospital 'where everything's taken care of.' A lot of people said to me that home birth was ridiculous, and why even consider it. (Murray)***

Several fathers said that the most vocal opposition to the idea of home birth often came from friends and relatives who had had children themselves. The apparent wisdom of these more experienced people can lend a sense of legitimacy to their views, even if these views are opposed to your own.

> ***What I found a bit worrying was that friends with children were saying, Don't be ridiculous, you can't do it at home and have no pain relief. They were quite openly mocking the idea, which is quite hard, because then it makes you question, Am I just being a bit of a hippie about this, thinking that we can do it all nice and liberal when the reality is going to be that it's a big mistake? It does put the doubts back into your head. (Bob)***

While your partner will try to cope with this opposition in her own particular way, this kind of conflict has a very particular kind of sting in its tail for you. Friends and family may see home birth as being solely your partner's idea and, as the man in the relationship, they may expect you to 'talk her out of it' or 'put your foot down'. Many people find it difficult to understand why birth choices matter so much to women, and they may have an even harder time understanding why you support these choices too. As Willie from

Scotland explains:

> *Most people said to me, 'You've got to change her mind on that, you can't let her do that at home – there's too much risk involved.' (Willie)*

When such comments come from your parents, your siblings or your closest friends, they establish an uncomfortable tug-of-war; on one side are the well-meaning doubters who expect you to put a stop to this 'foolish' idea of home birth; on the other, there's your partner, who needs and expects your support; and in the middle, you. It may be difficult for you to have your convictions put to the test in this way, especially if you have only just managed to overcome your own fears about home birth.

If you are experiencing opposition from those whose opinions you value the most, it may help you to put their comments into context. What kinds of thoughts and experiences have informed these negative attitudes? In many cases, it may be possible that your loved ones are voicing their concern not out of anger, but out of a genuine fear that you will end up having the kind of traumatic birth that they themselves have witnessed or experienced. Here, two fathers explore the rationale behind the comments made by their nay-saying relatives:

> *Generally, older relatives were against the idea, as they had been effectively 'forced' to have hospital births for their children in the '60s and '70s, with no realistic alternative being available. (David N.)*

> *People thought we were crazy. I remember clearly my brother-in-law saying, 'You don't know what you're doing, you'd better get into hospital, get it over and done with. Birth isn't a bed of roses, like you think it is'. My sister had had all sorts of complications during the birth of her daughter, she had laboured for 24 hours, the head had been fully engaged and she couldn't dilate enough, so she had to have a Caesarean. Later, on the night when our daughter was born safely at home, my sister and brother-in-law came round*

to the house. After hearing our story, they were both sitting on the couch crying. Both of them just thought it was the most wonderful thing compared to the experience they'd had. (John)

It may be disappointing to face hostility at the very point in your partner's pregnancy when you would like to feel confident and optimistic about your plans for a home birth, but as the stories above demonstrate, it is important to put such reactions into perspective. People are inevitably influenced by their own subjective experiences, and they are entitled to their opinions, just as you are entitled to yours.

The question remains: how will you build a positive attitude if and when those closest to you are convinced that you're making a terrible mistake? Some of them may be silenced or, at least, temporarily softened by statistics and research that demonstrate the safety of home birth. Others may be reassured if you remind them how close you are to the nearest hospital in the event of a genuine emergency. However, if certain people continue to remind you of your 'foolishness' at every opportunity, waving the proverbial red flag up until the very moment when your partner's waters break, then it may be best to follow a diplomatic tack and simply avoid the subject of birth as far as possible. In most cases, anti-home-birth rants can be brought to a close by a polite but firm assurance that you and your partner are happy to take responsibility for the informed choice that you've made together.

Of course, if you are utterly convinced that the people closest to you will react badly to your plans, then you and your partner might choose to avoid the conflict altogether by keeping your decision to yourselves until all has been said and done, as this Stuart from Scotland did:

We pretended that we were going to the hospital, and then called everyone with the good news afterwards – gleefully, and somewhat smugly.

How can we get some support as we plan for our home birth?

One of the best ways of establishing a positive support network during your partner's pregnancy is to seek out like-minded parents. If you've spent so much time justifying your birth choices to skeptical friends that you've begun to spout perinatal mortality statistics in your sleep, then you may be starting to feel like you're the only man ever to plan for a normal, joyful birth. Nothing could be further from the truth; if you look in the right places, you will find other men and women – be they first-timers or seasoned parents – whose hopes, fears, and birth choices are similar to your own.

Depending on the prevailing attitudes and resources in your region, you and your partner may be able to join a local home birth support group. In your mind, the words 'home birth support group' may conjure up a woodland hut where a hippie bouncer enforces a strict 'hempwear and sandals' dress code; you flash your new Birkenstocks and nervously enter the hut, where big-bellied women are gathered around a fire, trading tips on perineal massage in between choruses of 'No Woman No Cry'. If you would rather eat a bucket of hair than attend such a gathering, then think again – most of these groups are supportive, informal affairs run by parents who, themselves, have planned and experienced successful home births. Meetings are a chance to ask questions, share information, and gain moral support. The father to your left may be wearing a hemp tunic, but there's also a pretty decent chance that he'll look and feel a lot like you.

Even if there are no such groups in your area, there will almost certainly be a variety of antenatal classes. These classes may be offered by your local hospital or they may be privately run; in the UK, independent classes are offered by organisations such as the National Childbirth Trust and Birthlight, or by individuals who offer their own workshops, while in the US, there are countless classes for parents who want to learn birthing 'methods' such as Bradley, Lamaze, or Birthing From Within. Classes are usually geared towards first-time mothers and fathers, although 'refresher' courses are sometimes available for more experienced parents. The classes may be offered as a series of six or eight sessions, or they may take place over the course of a weekend. Regardless of the format, each class usually covers some combination of antenatal wellness, the physiological stages of labour, different forms of pain relief, and early parenting skills. Some classes may be based on a more conventional, medicalised approach to birth, while others may promote normal birth and encourage a degree of self-reflection.

If you and your partner would like to attend an antenatal class, it may be useful to consider exactly what you both hope to get out of such a class before actually choosing one. Are you mostly interested in the physical process of labour and birth? Do you want a class in which your role as a supporter will be explored and explained, or would father-focused discussions make you uncomfortable? Are you looking for an intimate environment in which to share your hopes and fears, or would you and your partner prefer to 'blend in' with a larger group? Will home birth be promoted as a viable option in your class, or will the group leader assume that all participants are heading for the hospital?

Men's experiences of antenatal classes appear to vary widely. Midwife and birth sociologist Rosemary Mander argues that, 'enlightened and well-meaning attempts to improve the man's position are doomed to failure' due to the prevalent confusion about the actual role of the man himself during pregnancy and birth.[2] However, some participants do express great satisfaction with their classes. Some men, like David N. from England, seem to appreciate them from a largely informational point of view:

> ***Our classes helped to prepare us for the actual birth, and the different stages of labour and how to cope with them. It was particularly useful to understand the different pain-reducing options at each stage and the consequences of using them. These classes were not specifically aimed at home birth or hospital birth although, interestingly, only two couples out of***

the ten present were planning on a home birth.

For other fathers, antenatal classes are a safe environment in which to explore and confirm their decision to birth at home:

> *The teacher was very sympathetic and had a very gentle approach to childbirth and, if anything, she was a little biased towards the natural side of birth. At the beginning we thought she was a little flaky, but as time wore on, we found out more about the medical processes you would have to go through if you had to go to hospital to have your baby. . . Before the antenatal classes, I thought home birth was a very hippie, backward thing to do, but I have a very different view about it now. (Chi)*

In recent years, birth educators have begun to realise that what fathers share among themselves may be vastly different from what they might contribute to a mixed group of men and women. As American father Jorge puts it,

> *We had a home visit from the midwife to answer mainly my questions, but I would have been more satisfied if I had heard the same information from an experienced dad. It's just a guy thing, wanting to identify with another guy's experience.*

To satisfy that need for peer support, many classes set aside times where men and women divide into groups for some candid discussion, and some classes are exclusively single-sex all the way through. You may be uncomfortable sharing your thoughts about birth with other men, particularly if you sense that your choice to have a home birth will be challenged or ridiculed by the group. However, when the group dynamic is positive, you may be able to explore your feelings with a degree of honesty that might not have been possible in your partner's presence. One father describes, in *Juno* magazine, how his antenatal course took him from skepticism to revelation:

The first session meant nothing to me and I grumbled all the way home. It was at the second session that I had my epiphany. [The instructor] asked the women to step outside for a while because she wanted a chat with the men. She probed and interrogated each of us until finally one of us broke and explained what he felt. It was fantastic for me to hear I was not alone with my trepidations, fears and feeling of isolation from the birth... I was a different man going home that night.[3]

This kind of transformative experience depends largely on the sensitivity and skill of the group leader, as well as the dynamic of the attending fathers. However, this father's comments demonstrate how some classes can result in real personal growth.

Whether your course is just for men or mixed, large or small, hospital-based or private, the right class may give you the confidence that you need to maintain a positive outlook.

Which books, magazines and websites should I be looking at?

When plans are being made for a home birth, knowledge is power. Certainly, the ability to make informed choices lies at the heart of many successful home birth stories, and you may have already embarked on a quest for information beyond the pages of this book. Thanks to the Internet, any father-to-be can access reams of clinical studies, personal anecdotes and cautionary tales as he and his partner prepare for their child's arrival. Not so long ago, many babies were named after the midwife into whose hands they slipped; now, many babies' births are so thoroughly researched on the Internet that the day can't be far away when kindergartens worldwide are filled with giggling Googles and cute little Yahoos. Venture away from your computer and wander down to your local newsstand, where the print media offers yet more information: you and your partner can pore over endless glossy pages offering 'expert advice' and 'labour suite secrets'.

As you and your partner have already worked so hard to establish and maintain a positive outlook, you might want to bear in mind that the media can have a powerful effect on your attitude. Whether you spend hours online or just minutes flicking through magazines, you are absorbing information that will – consciously or unconsciously – affect your thinking about the potential risks and benefits of your home birth. Knowledge may indeed be power, but as your knowledge about pregnancy, birth, and parenting grows, you may want to take time every now and again to evaluate which information has been useful and empowering, and which has been confusing or upsetting.

You and your partner may find it increasingly important to surround yourself with positive thoughts, images, and people as your baby's arrival approaches. As your confidence grows and your faith in each other deepens, your vision of a healthy, happy home birth is one step closer to becoming a reality.

3

Choosing the Guest List

Anyone present at a home birth is there by invitation only. Would you like to create a party atmosphere, with a dozen friends and relatives cheering on each contraction? Or would you prefer an aura of intimacy, with only yourself and your partner in the room? Either way, the choice is yours. As you begin to plan your home birth, it is important to consider who would enhance the experience and who might be, to put it kindly, surplus to requirements. Once you have chosen your guest list, you will be a step closer to visualising and achieving an event that has value and meaning for you, your partner and your new family unit.

What do midwives do, and how are they qualified to handle births without doctors?

In a culture where hospital birth is the norm, it may be difficult for you to imagine a birth without doctors. The doctor, gowned and masked, is an iconic authority figure: he controls the delivery room and all those who work and labour within it. He works in partnership with the clock on the wall, ensuring that birth progresses efficiently and quickly; when it does not, he intervenes with tricks and tools that only he is qualified to use. Now that you are planning a home birth, it may take time for you to usher this imposing figure into the wings of your imagination, and to welcome another player, the midwife, onto the stage.

Since the earliest days of humanity, women have attended other women in childbirth. The wisdom of midwifery is an ancient one: it is a wisdom that recognises and honours birth in all of its unpredictable glory, and one which celebrates the power of women to bring new life into the world. Until a few hundred years ago, it would have been unthinkable for most labouring women to be attended by a man, but the advent of such instruments such as forceps changed the balance of power in the birthing room forever. Michel Odent describes the introduction of obstetrics in seventeenth-century France:

> ***For the first time women were required to give birth lying on their backs, so that doctors could use their forceps more easily. Tradition has it that this practice began when Louis XIV had his mistress endure labor in this position so that he could have a better view of the birth of his child from his hiding place behind a curtain.***[1]

The dynamics of the birth space had changed irrevocably. Moreover, the event was made more convenient and appealing for male observers, both the forceps-wielding obstetricians and, in the case described above, the father lurking furtively behind the drapes. The preference for male birth attendants trickled down from the aristocracy to the middle classes and beyond; doctors rarely had as much birth experience as midwives, but they carried with them a very desirable prestige.

Modern obstetrics has grown in leaps and bounds since those early days – today's obstetricians receive highly specialised training in all of the latest technology and techniques – but women's bodies have remained the same. A newly qualified obstetrician will be familiar with a long list of possible pathologies and complications but, because that list has been learned in a hospital environment, he or she has probably witnessed precious few, if any, normal births. Enter, or should we say, *re-enter* the midwife.

Who is the midwife of today? She is an expert in normal birth but, apart from that defining characteristic, her identity is as diverse as the women she serves. Recently, a coalition of midwives' groups in the US attempted to outline what they call the Midwives Model of Care, which:

> *Monitors the physical, psychological, and social well-being of the mother throughout the childbearing cycle*
>
> *Provides the mother with individualized education, counselling, and prenatal care, continuous hands-on assistance during labour and delivery, and postpartum support*
>
> *Minimises technological interventions*
>
> *Identifies and refers women who require obstetrical attention*[2]

Midwives can acquire this range of expertise in a variety of ways. In the UK, midwifery is offered either as a three-year degree programme, or as an eighteen-month supplement to nursing training. Regardless of the mode of qualification, all working midwives in the UK must register with the Nursing and Midwifery Council, which sets and maintains standards of clinical practice. In the US, Certified Nurse Midwives (CNMs) are formally trained in nursing and midwifery (as their name would suggest); they may practice in hospitals, homes or birth centres; and they are licensed to prescribe medication in all 50 states. In contrast, Direct-Entry Midwives (DEMs) are not required to gain expertise as nurses, but they do learn to provide care throughout the childbearing cycle by engaging in apprenticeship, self-study, hands-on experience and specialised midwifery courses. Some DEMs gain licensure in specific states, while others achieve the title of Certified Professional Midwife (CPM), which indicates an adherence to the standards set by the North American Registry of Midwives. Those uncertified and unlicensed women who learn the craft of midwifery outside of the strictures of any formal programme are known variously as lay midwives, traditional midwives, or even 'granny midwives'. This traditional path is not legally recognised in some states in the US, in the UK, or in many other industrialised countries, but the aims of the lay midwife are the same as those of her certified counterparts in every country: to serve women and their families on the journey to parenthood and, perhaps most importantly, to do no harm.

In addition to recognition of the midwife's professional expertise, many people have recognised the less quantifiable, more spiritual aspect of midwifery. Some women see midwifery as an occupation, but some also think of it as a powerful vocation. American midwife Ina May Gaskin felt the calling in the 1970s, when she began delivering the babies of friends as they embarked on a cross-country trip in a convoy of old school buses. The group later settled in a kind of countercultural community in Summertown, Tennessee, known as the Farm, where Gaskin and some like-minded women set up their own midwife-led birth center. In her book *Spiritual Midwifery*, Gaskin describes the ethos that she and her Farm colleagues still follow to this day:

> ***The Vow of the Midwife has to be that she will put out one hundred percent of her energy to the mother and the child that she is delivering until she is certain that they have safely made the passage . . . The midwife must keep herself in a state of grace . . . A person who lives by a code that is congruent with life in compassion and truth actually keys in and agrees with the millions-of-years-old biological process of childbirth.***[3]

Lest you think this 'code' is a load of New Age mumbo-jumbo, it's worth noting that the birth center at The Farm has become internationally known and respected over the years for its outstanding record of safe, normal births. Passion and expertise need not be mutually exclusive.

While it is easy to see how midwife-led care can benefit mothers, the advantages for expectant fathers may be less immediately obvious. Many of the fathers who were interviewed for this book expressed their confidence in and satisfaction with the midwives who cared for their partners. You may wonder whether your midwife really 'knows her stuff'; one father says he was reassured by the competence of the midwives who attended his wife in labour, and by their apparent readiness to seek help if and when help was necessary:

> *In my profession [as a cardiac physiologist], I know the boundaries of what I can do and what I can't do in my job; for example, when to phone and get help in an emergency like a cardiac arrest. The midwives, the way they were checking, if there had been any problem I'm sure they would have told us whether we needed to go into hospital. Whatever they might say at the time, we were comfortable that they were within their boundaries, so we were happy that they knew what they were doing. Both of them were really good and really supportive. (Murray)*

A desire for continuity of care was also a recurring theme among home-birthing fathers:

> *By engaging [our midwife] directly, we had a caregiver that we had a one-to-one relationship with . . . I think that relationship is quite important because, getting back to the actual point of birth, everyone needs to know what the plan is and stick to it, and it's much better if it's the same people rather than just whoever's on duty at that time. (Rajiv)*

For Rajiv and others like him, midwifery care means the opportunity to create a team where every member plays a part in creating and implementing a positive birth plan. This continuity of care may be slightly harder to achieve if you are 'assigned' a team of midwives, as may be the case if you are in the UK and choose to book a home birth through the National Health Service. In that case, it is worth exploring your area's provisions for home birth; some community midwifery units are used to attending home births with enthusiasm and expertise, while others may be less outwardly supportive. If any member of your designated birth team is unsupportive of your partner's plans, then your partner is completely within her rights to request a replacement.

Wherever you are, you and your partner may wish to discuss the qualities you value the most in a midwife. Does your ideal midwife keep her training up to date? Does she stay calm under pressure? Is her sense of humour important to you? What kind of clinical back-up does she have, in case of emergency? Ultimately, any midwife you choose must be a trusted member of your birthing team; someone who will nurture and care for your partner; and someone who will honour and respect your role as a father-to-be.

What is a doula, and why should we think about having one at our birth?

You may have heard about doulas on television or in one of your partner's pregnancy magazines; perhaps friends have used doulas at their children's births and have recommended that you do the same. Who are these people with the exotic-sounding job title? What could they possibly bring to your team, and isn't their presence in the birth space just some kind of newfangled trend for middle-class parents with more money than sense?

Let's start with that crazy name. 'Doula' is an ancient Greek word for 'woman servant', and the term has been increasingly used over the past few decades to describe a woman, usually a mother herself, who offers practical, emotional and informational support to other women and their partners during the childbearing year. The role itself is much older than the name that it has been given in recent times. Quite apart from any clinical context, women have been supporting each other around the time of birth for as long as babies have been born. Most women were able to take this kind of continuous peer support for granted until just a few generations ago; now, many women in the industrialised West face birth as an isolated and isolating event. Many of them live far from their families, and even those that do have female relatives and friends nearby feel unable or unwilling to share the birth process with them.

The role of today's doula goes far beyond hand-holding. A doula usually meets with a woman several times during her pregnancy to discuss the woman's reproductive history, her general wellness, her hopes and fears for the birth, her choices in medical care, and any additional concerns about the transition to motherhood. During the birth itself, hand-holding can indeed play a prominent role, as does any other support the labouring mother requires. Doulas rub backs, make snacks, offer moral support, suggest positions and techniques to keep labour comfortable and efficient, and give partners breaks as and when breaks are needed. After the birth, the doula usually visits the new parents at home at least once, to discuss the birth, to offer support for feeding and, of course, to admire the new baby. Some doulas specialise in postnatal care and will visit on a regular basis for weeks or even months after the birth, providing more comprehensive feeding support and practical help around the home. It must be noted that, in addition to all the things that doulas do, their role is also defined by the one thing they won't do: they don't provide clinical care. A doula does not take a mother's blood pressure, perform internal examinations or deliver a baby. Instead, she works alongside the midwife, offering a different kind of care, but one which can be just as beneficial. Research attests to this benefit: the continous presence of a doula during birth has been shown to cut the average length of labour for first-time mothers, to decrease the need for analgesic pain relief such as epidurals, to lower a mother's chances of requiring a surgical delivery (i.e., forceps or Caesarean section), to increase a mother's satisfaction with the birth experience, and to reduce a mother's chances of developing postnatal depression.[4]

Facts and figures aside, many fathers are skeptical of the need for yet another member of the birthing team. If you are worried about a doula 'taking over' your role or controlling the birth, then you're not alone, as these fathers explain:

The first thing I thought when my wife said she'd bring in a doula was, 'What am I not giving you that someone else can? So I was a bit upset to start with but, again, I did research and found out about it, and then I met [the doula] and realised that she was someone Suzanne could go to, not just at the birth but throughout the whole process, keeping her on track and making sure she was mentally ready for the birth. She would be another trained person that Suzanne knew would be able to help, so that was great. (Murray)

I came into one of the sessions a bit sceptical, but when the doula came along and explained in her very gentle and supportive way how she would work, that did help. She was easy to like, and that was important to me. (Willie)

These fathers, and many others like them, came to realise that, rather than inhibiting their role as birth supporters, doulas actually facilitated their participation by relieving them of the enormous burden of being the sole birth 'coach'. Men may feel confident about learning relaxation techniques, dealing with medical caregivers, and staying calm in the face of challenges and complications but, on the birth day itself, even the most self-assured father may be overwhelmed by the intensity of the event. One father explains how he thought a doula might help him and his partner to stay calm during their child's birth at home:

We wanted someone on our team that could help and support with things like breathing techniques and relaxation techniques and things to keep my wife calm, perhaps better than I could. I'd read a lot about birth but was also aware that without having done it before, you don't know how you're going to react yourself and, in all truth, I could easily have freaked out and gone, 'Sorry, actually I can't help at all, I'm actually really tense.' We wanted someone who could help keep [my wife] in the state of mind she needed to be in. (Bob)

Another father explains how a doula offered welcome support with pain relief during his wife's labour:

> ***Julia needed constant back massaging throughout to help her get through the pain, and whenever she was in the birth pool, she had to have warm water slowly poured over her back. Be prepared to let your doula also provide support to your partner, especially through gentle touch and massaging. Get a good doula and it will help your home birth tremendously. (David N.)***

If your partner feels confident that you will be able to meet all of her needs during labour and birth, then a doula may not be for you. However, if either of you doubt your ability to be an all-seeing, all-knowing birth coach/father/lover/masseur, and if you would welcome the support of someone who can provide you both with a listening ear and a steady hand along your journey to parenthood, then doula support may be an option you might like to explore.

Chi's Story
A doula-supported birth

Chi is an engineer from Cambridge, England. He and his wife Sophie hired a doula for their son's birth at home. This story illustrates the practical and moral support that a doula can offer to both parentsr, especially during a long and difficult labour.

It all happened on Sunday night. It was after dinner, we were just settling down, and Sophie felt something and said, 'It's starting.' I got very excited and wondered whether we had everything ready, not realising it was going to be quite a long labour.

I made Sophie comfortable and tried to pamper her if she wanted this

or that, bringing her cups of tea and that sort of thing. At the beginning, because the early onset of labour wasn't too uncomfortable for her, I think she quite enjoyed the early bits. Then it sort of went through until the early hours of the morning.

The intensity – and the anxiety, I suppose – slowly built up, so it wasn't till about two or three o'clock in the morning that we called Maddie, the doula. She came for a bit in the early hours of the morning, she had a look and said everything was quite normal, and then she went away for a bit and came back later in the morning.

Sophie tried to rest a while and the labour went on to the following day. Everything was going quite normally, and then during the day things started to slow down again. To me, everything felt and looked normal. I didn't know any different, so I thought that people went through stages of repeating lulls and troughs. Little did I know that it was meant to be progressing. I later found out that Maddie had been quite concerned at that point because labour wasn't progressing – it had slowed down quite a lot, and Sophie was starting to get more and more tired. The day before, she had managed to have some rest, but at this point, she couldn't rest. We tried different things. Sophie went for a bath and things like that to relax, but that actually had an adverse effect.

On that second evening, at about eight or nine o'clock, the midwife came along. She said everything was quite normal – hunky dory. She was another one of those experienced midwives. Even if things weren't 100 percent right, she wouldn't show any serious concern; she was very calm and experienced, and we trusted her.

There were a lot of things going on by that time. I was going to get grapes for Sophie to suck on, and at one point she wanted some heat around her belly to help the pain, so I was running back and forth with hot towels and this little bean bag to heat up. It's quite strange because in between running around, I felt a bit like a spare, as far as husbands do. I didn't know what to expect; everything was new to me, but I didn't feel too badly off because this was my house, my home.

When active labour really started to happen, I tried helping Sophie to stand and sit, and that sort of thing. Maddie was great at that point; she made some suggestions as to what sort of positions Sophie should adopt. It ended up that she was quite happy leaning against the banister of the stairs.

There was one point when Sophie was leaning against Maddie for support. Maddie, being Maddie, said, 'Come over here, Chi, let Sophie lean on you,' and Sophie shouted, 'NO!!!' Sophie later said that at that point, she felt like what she needed was to have another woman around, not a man, even though that man was me. I can't remember whether I took offence at that, but certainly I was quite peripheral at that point.

It wasn't until right at the end that I got involved in the actual birth itself. I was sitting on the settee with Sophie sitting between my legs, leaning back against me. I was supporting her arms, and she squatted and gave birth that way. I felt very involved; however, I didn't get a view of the actual birth itself. I still regret to this day that I didn't actually see the birth, but at least I felt that I was part of the process, offering support. I was pleased about that.

Should our other children be present at the birth?

Imagine this scenario: it's three o'clock in the afternoon, and your partner is on all fours in the corner of the living room, breathing through the contractions that have been coming since the wee small hours of the morning. You are beside her, massaging her back with scented oils, whispering words of encouragement in her ear. Things are getting more intense, and the sunlight spilling through the window illuminates the sheer concentration on your partner's face as another surge builds deep inside her. Her brow furrows, she moans and bucks . . . and then the door to the hall swings open. Your three-year-old zooms into the room wearing nothing but a Superman cape and a mischievous grin. You've left a video on in his room, and from down the hall, you can hear Bob the Builder shouting instructions at his crew. 'I farted and a poo came out!' your son roars, and the mood is irrevocably broken.

Now, imagine a slightly different scene: it's three o'clock in the morning. The flames of a dozen candles cast a flickering glow on the walls of the living room, and the air is heavy with the fragrance of clary sage and lavender. Your partner is in the birth pool; she leans back in the water, her eyes close, and she forms a perfect circle with her lips as she blows away the last contraction. The midwife is there, shining a flashlight into the pool, and you are next to her, gazing in amazement at the tiny patch of your baby's head now visible beneath the water. Your son is there too, in his Spiderman pyjamas; he sits bolt upright in your lap, rapt with attention. As your partner gives one final push and your baby slips out into the water, your son begins to laugh, and the giggle is contagious. Your partner cuddles the slippery baby into her chest, laughing, crying, delighted with her family.

For some women, having another child or children around during labour would be an unthinkable distraction. However, if you already have a child and are thinking about welcoming him or her into the birthing space this time around, you may well wonder which one of the scenes described above might be closer to reality. The answer is either one, potentially. Having an older child or children at a home birth can be a tremendously special event in the life of your family, or it can be a misjudgment that results in frustration and distress for all concerned.

Some people feel strongly that excluding children from the birth space has negative repercussions on them, on the family unit, and even on society as a whole. Sheila Kitzinger is an advocate for children's participation:

> ***All of us who approach childbirth with no experience of it, no idea of what happens except what can be gained from books and films, are in some sense deprived... In medicalising childbirth and removing it from the home, in separating it from the family, our culture has made birth, like dying, a fearful ordeal that can be dealt with only by trained experts, that is no longer part of our shared lives, and is out of women's control. In bringing birth back into a setting that is controlled by women, making it a family occasion, and involving the children, we reclaim it, and prepare children to reclaim it for themselves later in their own lives.***[5]

You may or may not agree with Kitzinger, but regardless of your perspective, you will still need to consider the basic practicalities of accommodating your older child or children at your home birth, especially since you may be the one to bear the brunt of the childcare while your partner gets on with the business of labour. Pat Thomas urges parents to take a pragmatic approach:

> ***Be realistic about your child. Don't expect a toddler to be immediately moved or transformed by labour and birth... Be prepared for your child to need someone to wipe a bottom or a nose, to be hungry or grumpy, to say 'no', to argue and fuss, to need cuddling and want to show you something or know where their favourite Teletubbies video is.***[7]

Labour can be shockingly short or mind-bendingly long; if you choose to make birth an all-family event, it pays to think about how you will entertain, comfort, and support your older child or children in either case.

Age alone may not be an adequate indicator of your child's readiness to witness labour and birth. A very young child may be able to participate in the event with surprising maturity; by contrast, an older sibling may be overcome by unexpected emotion or overtaken by boredom. The following questions may be useful as you and your partner discuss whether your child is likely to be a party crasher, or a guest of honour:

Would you like your child to be present for the whole labour or just the final stages of the birth?

Does your child understand the basic facts about what happens during labour and where the baby actually comes from?

Is your child likely to be able to cope with the sights and sounds of the birth space; will his/her mother's efforts upset him/her?

Your own attitude towards birth will have enormous influence on your child's demeanour at the event. Are you capable of providing your child and your partner with calm, confident support, or are you likely to communicate feelings of stress and fear?

How are you likely to behave if there are unexpected challenges or complications?

You and your partner know your child better than anyone else; you must make the choice based on sensitive considerations of his or her personality.

Jorge's Story
When Mommy's a midwife

Jorge is a videographer from Ithaca, New York, and his wife, Monica, is a midwife. In the story below, their daughter Taina plays a supportive role during the home birth of her little brother.

My wife, Monica, is a home birth midwife, so there was never any question as to where we were going to have the births. My wife chose a midwife colleague to just observe, and jump in only if necessary. We also had her mother, the nurse / friend that works with my wife, and our four-year-old daughter, Taina.

Monica started having contractions right after dinner at 7p.m.. We called the midwife and the nurse right away. We had our own Jacuzzi in the front porch, and Monica relaxed there for a while. Taina kept coaching her, 'You're doing great, Mommy, just breathe,' and she also massaged Monica continuously.

We decided to set up in the living room because it was centrally located to everything that we needed. I was on the edge of the couch holding Monica from behind. It was excruciating for me to hold her in that position, but I knew that she was going through so much more pain than I was. Meanwhile, my mother-in-law was attending to Taina. It was amazing that my daughter was present for the entire labour and birth. I know that it will have a life-long positive effect on our daughter.

Monica began pushing at one point, but what came out was poop. We were all surprised, and Monica was a little embarrassed, but we all just encouraged her to keep going. The baby came out shortly afterwards. When the baby was on Monica's chest, again it was a soothing and sweet smell. Monica touched the baby, and found out that this time we had a boy. I remember jumping for joy, screaming, 'I have a boy, I have a boy!' Then I looked at my daughter, and said, 'Now I have a girl, and a boy!'

Afterwards, we just relaxed and continued calmly. There's nothing more rewarding for your family than a birth gone right! No regrets, no interventions, immediate skin to skin connection, and your wife feeling completely empowered.

Geoff's Stories

A family grows at home

Geoff is an American academic and father of four who feels strongly about the importance of birth as a family event. Here, he describes the births of two of his children, both of which were attended by older siblings.

My wife and I were introduced to the idea of home birth when we were preparing for the birth of our first child. In our circle of new expecting parents, some were considering home birth, and they shared with us some of the particulars of the preparation. We were also fortunate enough to have seen some home births on video in our birth classes. While not opposed to the idea, we didn't feel like it was something we were interested in pursuing.

We ended up having one hospital birth and then one birth-centre birth, and then when we were preparing for the birth of our third baby, my wife was very eager to have a different experience. She and I both felt very confident about the process of labour and the health of our babies. In addition, after the birth of our second child, my wife had become a certified birth instructor. In the course of her training, home birth was shown to be as safe as hospital birth for low-risk pregnancies.

So, when it was time to give birth a third time, we actively pursued birth practitioners who would provide a home birth; she wanted to be attended to by midwives rather than doctors. There's also something to giving birth in the home that connects you and your child to the house, to the street, the neighborhood, and the community. It also is a chance for the older siblings to connect with the new baby by being present at the birth.

First, the story of Candelaria, our third child: I showed up at home after work one evening, and my wife greeted me with a contraction. We sat down to dinner with our two sons and a friend who was visiting. After dinner, our friend put the children to bed while we went upstairs to fill the birth tub. This turned out to be a waste of time, although we did try a few contractions in it as it was filling up.

We attempted to get in touch with the midwife, but her answering service was not operating correctly. At this point, our confidence in the home birth ebbed a bit, since we hadn't contemplated the question of 'What if she doesn't show up?' We moved from the tub into a warm shower, and I alternated holding my wife with checking the phone and trying to call the midwife again.

We eventually got a hold of her, and she made her way to our house. We were relieved, but the contractions were getting quite painful. I think we were in the shower for nearly two hours, but miraculously, the hot water never ran out. The midwife came into the bathroom to evaluate Maria, at which point we went to the bedroom down the hallway that was set up for the birth.

We laboured a bit on the bed, and I could tell from what Maria was saying that she was nearing transition. Soon, she felt the urge to push, though it was a little more painful than she anticipated. At the midwife's suggestion, she changed position, at which point the water broke. This was a great relief, and the pushing started in earnest after this. Not too much longer, it was clear the baby was nearly out. We sent my wife's niece and friend to wake our boys from their beds so they could witness the birth. Our younger son wanted to, but our older son was a little scared. My wife's friend stayed in the bedroom with him, and they listened to the birth, rather than watching it.

The baby came out so quickly. The midwife toweled her off before giving her to my wife to nurse. We then cut the cord and held our baby, Candelaria, until morning.

In my wife's pregnancy with our fourth child, Calliope, we had just switched midwives at 42 weeks after feeling unsupported by our previous midwife. My wife had completed a second acupuncture treatment [to start the labour], but we felt our time was running out. We came home and had dinner with the kids. Then we put them to bed, I with the boys and Maria with our daughter. After they were asleep, we met in the hall, and Maria was feeling contractions. We didn't want to be fooled, but we were so excited, we couldn't contain ourselves.

We waited a bit until calling our friends (this was about nine or ten in the evening), who came over right away to help out. This time, some of our friends helped in the relaxation and pain relief. One new approach, which my wife thought of in between contractions, was to generate counterpressure with a piece of fabric wrapped and tightened around her hips. This was a great help as labour progressed.
When the midwives arrived (two plus one apprentice), we were moving between the bathroom and the bedroom. The shower was not as helpful this time as it was last time. We made it to the bed, fortunately, though we had to stop a couple of times and kneel on the floor. It was definitely a more painful birth than the previous one.

The overall mood was one of encouragement. There was a unity of spirit among all the attendants. One thing I noticed was that although our friends were extremely helpful, they still had a tiny amount of fear in their eyes. When the midwives arrived, I think that fear disappeared. What they brought besides all their equipment and expertise was a very real sense that this labour was not in any way unusual or potentially dangerous. This was communicated to us both verbally but also by their attitude.

The midwives were very unobtrusive; you could tell they really trusted Maria's body to lead the way. Maria's friends and I helped relieve her pain a bit, but it was clear she was in transition. When it was time to push, we knew it wouldn't take long. We sent some of Maria's friends upstairs to fetch the children (it was now around midnight). This time, they all wanted to stay and watch, though it must have felt like a dream to them. We had prepared them by watching some of my wife's instructional birth videos, and we had always talked about birth in this non-mysterious way, but I think being confronted with the living reality is still hard to prepare for.

Calliope emerged very quickly and she was so healthy, with the exception of the cord wrapped slightly around her neck. The midwife effortlessly unhooked her and placed her at Maria's breast. Our son was eager to cut the cord when it was time.

Eventually, the kids returned to bed after a few rounds of board games, and the midwives cleaned up. When we woke up in the middle of the night, we realised that it was just the six of us in the house. It occurred to us that it was just our family in this house, and that this family now included a baby just hours old. The house seemed emptier and bigger than it had been before the birth. But it, and our family, seemed more complete.

What about friends and family at the birth?

In many cultures, children aren't the only possible guests at a birth; friends, neighbours and relatives weave in and out of the birth space, some offering soft words of encouragement, some preparing sweet snacks to nourish the labouring mother, and some simply bearing silent witness to the power of birth. In our modern, industrialised society, we are used to a slightly different birthing circle: just mother, father, and a team of specialised medics. Home birth offers you the flexibility to expand or contract this circle as much as you'd like; you and your partner might wish to keep the event intimate and private, or you might like to create a vibrant atmosphere, with a band of well-wishers providing constant support.

It is important to consider not only what a midwife, a doula or a child will bring to the birth, but also what any additional guests might contribute to the event. Casual remarks and furrowed brows that might not be noticed under normal circumstances can have significant effects on labouring women who, by the very nature of their task, must lay themselves bare to the emotions of the day. Will your partner take solace in the arms of her dear Aunt Gert, or will she be annoyed by Gert's heavy perfume and 'distinctive' laugh? Will you be glad of the support offered by the women from your partner's drumming circle, or will you be tempted to toss their bongos out the window after the umpteenth percussive rendition of 'We Shall Overcome'? Geoff, whose story is featured above, explains how he and his wife chose birth guests who would support their choices:

> ***I think in both [home birth] cases, my wife was very careful to consider who would be most useful in helping her keep her mental 'game' during labour. Two of her friends are prenatal yoga instructors, and all have had, or tried to have, natural childbirths. As for her sister, she has been at every birth, including the first one in the hospital. In a way, she was a reminder that we had done this before, and that we could do it again.***

By the time your partner goes into labour, you and she will have put a great deal of thought into your decision to have a home birth. As Geoff describes, anyone else who is privileged enough to be invited to the event must also have faith in birth as a normal, natural event that can occur safely at home. If Aunt Gert has the fire department, the paramedics, and your local obstetrician on speed dial, then she may not be the most confident member of your birth team.

What if we don't want anyone with us at the birth – not even a midwife?

The midwife, the doula, your children, your friends, your neighbours, your family . . . with a guest list this long, you may be starting to wonder whether you'll need to hire caterers and a marquee to accommodate your home birth team. Some parents choose to avoid such a dilemma by making their child's birth as intimate and private as possible. The only people on their guest list are the parents themselves. A home birth without a midwife is known as an unassisted birth, or freebirth, and the popularity of such births is growing around the world.

Parents come to the decision to freebirth from many different paths. Laura Shanley, author of *Unassisted Childbirth* and perhaps the most outspoken advocate of this practice, discusses how she and her husband, David, decided on freebirthing the first of their five children:

David had been researching birth trauma when he came across Grantly Dick-Read's book, *Childbirth Without Fear.* The book had a tremendous impact on him:

> ***When we decided to have a baby a few years later, we realised that if we gave birth with a doctor or midwife present, we would basically have to educate them about what we believed were the true causes for the problems in birth: interference and fear. Unassisted birth seemed like the best choice***

for us. At that time we were also reading books about the power of the mind. We felt confident that by visualising and believing in a safe and easy birth, we could create one.

David Shanley suggests that in addition to the benefits for mother and child, freebirthing gives men the chance to be intimately involved in birth:

In a freebirth, a father can truly participate physically, emotionally, and spiritually. When a midwife or doctor is involved, generally the father is pushed aside. Freebirth offers a father a rare opportunity to bond with his partner and children in ways he can barely imagine. It is truly a life-changing experience.

For the Shanleys, freebirthing was the ultimate leap of faith: faith in a woman's ability to deliver her child safely, and faith in the power of positive thinking. Another father, Brian from the US, talks about freebirthing as an expression of his love for his family:

No one knows how to care for my family better than I do, as a father. If you really care for your loved ones, you wouldn't let some random person in a hospital put them under knife and needle when nature has made us perfect to handle all the workings of how our children came to be.

This theme of the self-sufficient family unit is common among freebirthing parents. As Kim from Canada explains, 'For some time, I have had a desire to be self-sufficient by doing things on my own (building things, growing a garden, etc.). This seemed to fit into that nicely.' Still other parents choose unassisted childbirth as a last resort after being consistently disappointed by their antenatal care; they feel that 'going it alone' would be preferable to being attended in labour by representatives of a system that has already failed them. There are also a number of people who consider the act of freebirthing to be a testimony of their religious faith; they believe that God will guide the birth to safety.

If your mental alarm bells are ringing, you're not alone. While some parents choose freebirthing as the ultimate demonstration of their faith and love, many people see unassisted childbirth as the ultimate act of irresponsibility. The looming question of 'What if something happens?' is amplified a hundredfold in the absence of skilled birth attendants; it's easy to wonder how Mr. and Mrs. Joe Average could be prepared for the many obstetric challenges and complications that may arise when birth doesn't go to plan. Writing in the journal *Midwifery Today,* American midwife Ina May Gaskin suggests that 'approximately 10-15 percent of all births will require skilled assistance to reach a healthy outcome for mother and baby,' and she recalls several instances where mothers who had planned to freebirth either sought a midwife at the last minute, or died from unexpected complications. Freebirthing parents often argue that they will know when professional help becomes necessary during labour, but Gaskin goes on to argue that

> ***... some [women] are unable to have an objective view of what's happening with their bodies (especially when they are giving birth for the first time) and may lack the experience to distinguish true intuition from wishful thinking or outright delusion.***[7]

Clinical research isn't much clearer on the subject of unassisted childbirth. Several studies suggest that problems are more likely to occur in home births that are unplanned and unsupported by skilled caregivers.[8,9,10] Freebirthing advocates would argue that their home births are planned, and that the parents have often taken it upon themselves to become 'skilled' on both a practical and spiritual level. Here, Kevin from the US discusses his own careful preparations for an unassisted birth:

> ***I have to point out that this was not an act of irresponsibility. We had***

emergency measures in place. We had all of the supplies needed for the birth and maintained a sterile environment. We did all of the prenatal checks and carefully watched for signs of potential complications, we were pre-registered at the nearby hospital and had all of the emergency numbers handy and we were prepared to transfer to the hospital at any sign of possible complications.

Kevin and others like him are adamant that their freebirths are actually supported by careful contingency plans. However, research has failed to produce any substantial evidence of such conscientious preparation. Because this way of birthing is such a personal and relatively unusual choice, it would be impossible to conduct a randomised, controlled trial of the outcomes of freebirth versus planned, midwife-attended home birth. In the meantime, parents who are interested in 'going it alone' will have to rely on their own intuition and on the anecdotal evidence of other couples who have welcomed their babies in this way.

The legal status of freebirthing is nearly as confusing as its medical feasibility. In America, fear of prosecution has driven some freebirthing parents 'underground'; One father says,

I felt I needed to be guarded about my decisions, since people think [unassisted childbirth] isn't in the child's best interest in our area, and that it's something to notify the Department of Social Services about. (Brian)

British freebirthers inhabit a similarly grey area of the law. Jacqui Smith MP, a Minister of State for the UK Department of Health, attempted to clarify matters in a letter to another Member of Parliament, dated September 23, 2002:

Attending a woman in childbirth, as opposed to general support given by partners and relatives, has been an offence against the protected function of midwifery since the Midwives Act 1902 and the fines [a maximum of

£5000] are set at a level to reflect the seriousness of the offence. By 'attend' we mean, 'assume responsibility for care' and this is not intended to outlaw husbands, partners and relatives whose presence and support during childbirth are extremely important.[11]

For the freebirthing husband or partner, the line between 'attending' the mother of his child and 'assuming responsibility for [her] care' may be a fuzzy one. He is not impersonating a midwife, but neither is he a passive observer of the birth process. Some British freebirthing fathers get around this problem by phoning a midwife when they know the baby's birth is so imminent that the midwife will not possibly arrive in time; in this way, the parents safeguard their privacy while also appearing to have requested medical help. Some parents may be uncomfortable with this deception. For them, true peace of mind can only be achieved if the father keeps his hands firmly off the birth and the mother 'catches' the baby herself. In her book *Am I Allowed?*, Beverly Beech insists, 'The woman herself cannot be prosecuted for birthing her own baby – whatever and however she chooses to do it. There is no offence in law. If anyone tells you there is, they are misinformed, ignorant or lying.'[12]

Jeroen's Story
A family freebirth

Jeroen is a consultant and lecturer in Nijmegen, the Netherlands. After their first son, Thijn, was born in the hospital and their second son, Noek, was born at home with a midwife, Jeroen and his wife chose to go it alone for their third and final birth.

It is Wednesday, February 27th, 2008, seven o' clock in the morning. I wake up alone in our big family bed; I don't work on Wednesdays, and Wendy has already gotten up with Thijn and Noek. Wendy has been pregnant for more than 40 weeks now; she's a couple of days past her due date. We have planned to do this birth ourselves without professional help – no midwife, just the two of us. Eventually, I have become completely confident that we can do it.

The sun shines through the curtains and I step out of bed. In the bathroom, I notice Wendy has turned the heating on, which she never usually does, but that doesn't ring a bell with me yet. When I come downstairs, Wendy's sitting at the table with the boys. I see something in her face – she looks happy. Wendy tells me that her waters broke. It's about to begin!

Wendy doesn't feel any contractions during these first hours and we begin the day quietly and easily. After breakfast, I go with the boys to the supermarket. On our list are a lot of delicious things: fresh fruit juice, mangos, pears, ingredients for the steak salad I want to make for dinner tonight. It's a beautiful day, mild in temperature, and the sun shines.

When the boys and I get back from our shopping, the four of us have lunch together, and after that, Wendy goes upstairs. She'll stay on the bed all afternoon, having contractions in a relaxed way. I expect this to take all day and that the baby will be born at night, when Thijn and Noek are sleeping.

It's a perfect day, the sun is still shining, and the boys and I go into the garden. Thijn and Noek play in the sand and I'm drinking coffee in the sun. Meanwhile, Wendy is on our bed, taking a rest, reading a book, and every once in a while she has a contraction. She has a wonderful, quiet and relaxed afternoon, all alone on the bed. I make mango lassis with the boys and, at four o'clock, I take them for another trip, this time to the library. I still don't feel any need to hurry; Wendy and I feel that the birth will take place later on at night.

I come back from the library at five o'clock, and of course, I am eager to know how Wendy is doing, so I go upstairs. Wendy tells me the contractions are getting stronger. She wants to go in the bath, but she also wants to have dinner with us downstairs. So, I go down and start to make something special and easy: a salad of steak, mango, and watercress. While I'm making dinner, Wendy lets me know that she won't eat downstairs; she wants to go in the bath to handle the contractions. First, though, she sends an e-mail to the unassisted-childbirth mailing list, to let the women on the list know how everything is going. She had sent some e-mails earlier during the day and we feel that the women on the list are with us now. Wonderful!

It's 5.30pm. I bring some of the salad to Wendy in the bath, in case she wants to eat something. The salad is not a good idea. Wendy is having the final contractions of the dilation phase, and they are tough. She's calm, but I can see it's not easy for her. Things are going to happen fast now. I go downstairs and tell the boys, who are sitting at the table, ready for dinner, that the baby will be born soon and that I have to be with Wendy. I tell them that they can do what they want, what feels right for them. They both come upstairs with me.

I kneel down next to the bath, and Thijn and Noek stand close by as well. Wendy hasn't got much space to move around and that makes the contractions painful. It's tough for her, changing position is impossible, and getting out of the bath is totally out of the question now – it's too late for that. I am with Wendy, one hand on her forehead, one hand on her chest. I see that she is doing great, and I tell her that. I have no sense of time, but I know things are going fast. After the final contractions of the first stage, Wendy starts feeling the urge to push. She just follows the forces in her body, and her body is doing fine.

I can see now that Wendy is afraid of something. Later, she tells me that it was the fear that she wouldn't know what to do after the baby was born. I sit next to her and comfort her, make her feel at ease. It works and Wendy's fear disappears. Then the baby's head is going to be born. I see the head coming out and also sliding back in again. I can tell Wendy what's going on, and that corresponds with what she feels is happening. That gives Wendy strength. Everything is going fine.

Thijn sees the head being born; he and Noek have both been quiet and at ease the whole time. After the head, the first shoulder is born, and I really have to look hard to know what I'm seeing. It's a shoulder, a piece of an arm, and a lot of vernix. * *On the fifth push, the baby slides out of Wendy, into the water. My hands had been in the water all the time, feeling the head, and now I can catch the baby. I take my own child in my own hands! At that time, I am completely in the moment. Later, I realised that this moment was probably the most beautiful of my life.*

The baby is purple, but that doesn't scare me. There is a cry, and in a flash, I think, 'It breathes!' When I give the baby to Wendy, I think I see a little penis, but no, that's the umbilical cord. In the same look, I see that our baby is a girl. Surprised, happy, and confused, I say to Wendy, 'Wen, it's a girl!' Wendy takes her from me and lays her to her breast. So beautiful and simple: Roos is born!

Thijn and Noek are still standing next to us. The boys look a little overwhelmed at their sister. Now that she's born, they start moving again, walking from the bathroom to the other rooms, back and forth. We hear Thijn saying to Noek: 'Noek, it's a little sister!'

---

* *Author's note:* Vernix is the paste-like coating that protects a baby's skin in the womb.

When Wendy steps out of the bath, half an hour after Roos is born, the placenta is born. The five of us go to the bedroom, where I've made a place for us on the big family bed. We sit down and take a good look at Roos. She is so small, but she looks good and healthy. After a while, Wendy wants more freedom to move around and we cut the umbilical cord, which has gone completely white by that time. We put a little clamp near Roos's belly. This all feels like a completely normal and simple thing to do – probably the easiest part of the whole birth. Oddly enough, this is the thing most people ask about when we tell that Roos was born with only us present: 'How did you do that with the umbilical cord?' Well, exactly the same as the midwife would do it: clamp it and cut it!

Later on, Wendy looks at the placenta for a while to see if the placenta had come out completely. It looks perfect; no pieces have been left in her uterus. In the meanwhile, the five of us are sitting on our bed. I had taken the remains of dinner upstairs and so, we're still eating some of the wonderful salad. Wendy happily drinks some mango lassi, and Roos is also feeding well. Wendy has had trouble with breastfeeding in the past, but here, without any strange hands, nobody telling us what to do, everything goes so smoothly. Like it should, of course.

After a while, Thijn says it's time for beschuit *with* muisjes, *a typical Dutch tradition. A great idea! When a baby is born, you serve* beschuit, *crisp large biscuits, with* muisjes, *sugared aniseeds, on top. For a boy, the mice are blue and white; for a girl, pink and white. We stocked up on both of the colours. I get everything from downstairs and this is how we eat the first of many beschuiten, on the bed, crumbs covering the blankets. Our family has changed profoundly, and from the first moment, we're all completely in love with Roos.*

I am glad and grateful that I looked all my fears in the eyes and took the great jump into the unknown and unpredictable. We let Roos's birth happen the way it would. And that turned out to be the great start of a new life.

Brian's Story
Not your average freebirther

Brian is a US Marine from Newport, North Carolina. He defies the stereotypical image of a hippie, radical freebirthing dad, and here he tells the story of his daughter's amazing birth.

It was a cold sunny day when my wife went into labour. I remember her waking up throughout the night to sit in the bathtub. She woke up early and told me she'd be fine with just sitting in the tub for a while, but around eight o'clock she came in to drag me out of bed, because I'd thought she would be fine like she said and I'd gone to sleep. In a daze, I caught my wits and gathered myself. I cleared a comfortable spot on the couch and laid down a plastic sheet with some white cotton sheets over the top so she wouldn't have that sticky plastic against her skin anywhere. I was thinking about what I'd need during the birth, so I made a bucket of warm water and had a towel and a wash cloth; all this was done while tending to my wife as she had her contractions.

She had read somewhere that stimulation of the nipples was a good way to calm her from the pain of the contractions. Personally, I think she just needed some sort of distraction to steer her mind away from the pain, so I held her up, kneeling behind her, massaging her nipples, and she's just screaming and nothing's happening really. In between her contractions, I would talk to her and fill her glass with water. She would throw up the water and scream back at me. It was intense.

My most clear memory was when her water broke and she said, 'I'm just going to push and the baby's going to come soon, I can feel it.' It really wasn't too messy the whole time, she only bled a little before the baby's head came out.

The second I saw her head, I felt the biggest blow of emotion. It was love, fear, happiness, sadness, complete joy and just an overwhelming feeling of adrenaline rush. When Dorothy's head came out I kept my hand underneath it so as to catch her, and she came out so fast that I thought I would drop her. I didn't drop her. She was wet with fluid and so very beautiful.

I unravelled the umbilical cord, handed the yelling baby to my wife, and she nursed. I didn't know what else to do but laugh, cry, and kiss my wife. It was the single most invigorating experience in my life. I commenced to cleaning up my wife's body and then later dabbing the blood and fluid off of my baby's body.

I would say that if there was any way a baby was to be born, then being born in the middle of winter, in the middle of the living room, was best for us, and most definitely the most comfortable place. I have everything I need within my grasp inside my own house and I don't have to worry about someone taking the baby away from my wife to clean her up.

Whether you choose to have a guest list of one, two, four, or twelve, you and your partner will need to think carefully about the structure of your birthing team. What role will each participant play? What are your hopes and fears about each person's involvement? And perhaps, most crucially, how can you and your partner meet each other's needs during this most special of family events?

4

Pleasure and Pain

'The pain of childbirth has a bad reputation.'
Janet Balaskas

Imagine that your baby is about to arrive. Your partner is experiencing the most physically and emotionally overwhelming event of her life. As her pelvic ligaments stretch, her uterus contracts and the mouth of her womb eases open, great waves of sensation wash over her body. She feels conflicting urges to control these waves but also to surrender to them. As the pressure builds within her, so does a feeling of intense release. In the comfortable surroundings of her own home, and nurtured by the love of her man, pain is only the beginning of what your partner can experience during childbirth. Her contractions may test the limits of her endurance but, in between these surges, she may also withdraw into moments of blissful rest. Away from intravenous drips and ticking clocks, you can support your partner in experiencing labour in all of its awesome, challenging power.

For many fathers, the prospect of seeing their partners in unmedicated pain is the most daunting part of home birth. Without access to an epidural – referred to by some of its staunchest supporters as 'the happydural' – these men wonder how their partners will cope with labour and, also, how they themselves will respond to their partners' discomfort. Perhaps you share these concerns and, as you have never experienced childbirth, you might imagine that your partner will feel the kind of pain that you have felt during past episodes of injury or illness, perhaps a broken leg, a kidney stone, gastric flu or worse. You might think that each contraction will bring a longer, harder, stronger wave of this pain, peaking with the kind of bloodcurdling screams that are so prevalent in the labour wards of hospital dramas and films. Your heart races, you hide your eyes, and you wonder briefly whether you or your partner will pass out first.

It might be tempting to look for ways of 'fixing' this pain. After all, it's upsetting to see your partner struggling with such powerful sensations, and it's frustrating not to be able to stop this force that has taken control of her body. Patrick Houser is the director of Fathers-to-Be, an organisation that works with men as they prepare for parenthood, and he makes the following observation about men's response to labour pain:

> ***A man, typically, wants to immediately fix whatever is not to a woman's liking. Most men have what I call the 'fixing gene'. It has not been proved yet by science, however the anecdotal evidence is overwhelming. Fixing is not necessarily what is always called for.***[1]

In order to understand why contractions are not problems that need to be 'fixed', it is helpful to understand how and why they happen, as well as the benefits that their unimpeded progress can bring.

The sensations of labour are different from the 'dangerous' pain of illness and injury, in terms both of their origin and their effect. 'Dangerous' pain is your body's way of telling you that something is wrong, a kind of physical alarm bell caused by acute injury or illness. However, the labouring woman is neither sick nor injured, and the contractions that will eventually bring her baby to the outside world are caused by a hormone unlike any other, oxytocin. Oxytocin is the same hormone that is produced by the body when a person is in love, when he or she achieves sexual orgasm, and when a mother breastfeeds her child. In a normal, undisturbed, physiological birth, a steady tide of oxytocin floods the mother's body until it reaches its peak in the moments just after birth, encouraging mother and baby to bond in a moment of unparalleled intimacy. Any attempt to mask the pain of labour by artificial means also has the potential to diminish the positive effects of this oxytocin tide, as Janet Balaskas, the founder of the Active Birth movement, explains:

> ***Women talk of great ecstasy and bliss, of the deepest feelings of joy and love. It is important to realise that the pain involved is only part of the great variety of intense feelings one experiences. If one cuts out the pain one generally cuts out, to some extent, the other feelings too.***[2]

Thus, while your headache might benefit from a few aspirin and the pain of your broken arm could do with something a bit stronger, the sensations your partner will experience in labour require a bit more careful consideration.

This is not to say that home birth has to be an intensely painful ordeal if it is to be successful. On the contrary, there are a number of low-intervention techniques that can help your partner to stay as comfortable as possible during labour. You and your partner may have a natural affinity for certain relaxation techniques. For example, if you often massage each other as a way to unwind and get intimate, then you might find this to be an easily adaptable technique for pain relief during labour. Some interventions, like the use of a TENS machine, may be new to you and might require a bit more forethought. This chapter will explore some of the comfort measures your partner can use during labour, as well as your role in providing them. As you plan your journey to home birth, you might be reassured to know that nature has provided you with an arsenal of tricks and tools that can be just as effective as those offered by a hospital.

How can I create a birth space where my partner feels comfortable and calm?

Where would you rather have an orgasm? Would you rather be on a hospital bed, with bright fluorescent lights overhead, a ticking clock on the wall, and strangers observing your every movement? Could you still reach your peak if you were strapped to a beeping machine that monitored the speed, size, and intensity of your erection in second-by-second detail? Or would you be more likely to experience ecstasy in the comfort and privacy of your own home, with dimmed lights, familiar smells, and your favourite music playing softly on the stereo? If you chose the latter setting, then you're halfway to understanding why your partner's labour can be more comfortable and efficient at home than it might be in hospital. Oxytocin – the 'hormone of love' – flows more freely in an environment of undisturbed intimacy. This is not to say that a home birth will guarantee your partner a mid-labour orgasm (although a lucky few women do experience that phenomenon). However, the right surroundings can help your partner reap the benefits of oxytocin's effects during childbirth: regular, efficient, manageable contractions.

Here's where you come in. While your partner focuses on the final stages of her pregnancy and looks ahead to the birth of your baby, you can begin to think about ways of creating a comfortable birth space in your home. Women may always have supported other women in labour, but the role of men as creators of the birth space appears to be just as deeply embedded in human history. Whether it's Native Americans crafting birth supports from timber on the Great Plains or indigenous tribesmen building birth huts for their wives in Southeast Asia, fathers around the world have long embraced this practical role.[3] Don't worry if chopping wood and building huts isn't quite your thing; special birth spaces can be easily created in modern homes, too, as these fathers explain:

> ***We moved a sofa through to the dining room and covered it in old blankets. Suzanne wanted it to be like a nest where she could go and be quiet and keep warm. That was the idea, to have the nest there and to move between the birth pool and the nest, and when the baby was born, they could get warm and snuggle in there. (Murray)***

It was my job to set up the living room, move furniture, set up the pool, get out the towels and plastic sheets to protect the floor, etc. Together, we got the ambiance of the room just right – soft music playing, low lighting, and essential oils scenting the air. This was our living room – comfortable, familiar – home. The perfect place to have our baby. What a far cry from the hospital environment with its harsh lights, ammonia smells, and restricted visiting times. (Dan)

Like Murray and Dan, you can help make your partner's ideal birth space a reality. There is no need to redecorate your home completely. Often, simple touches, such as soft cushions, scented candles and gently opening flowers can be remarkably effective in creating a space where your partner can feel safe and uninhibited. Think about ways that your partner will use the space: is there a particular room in your home where she usually goes to relax and where she might be likely to spend most of her labour? Do you have any bean bags, stools or comfortable chairs that would help your partner adopt a variety of different positions? Up until now, you may have imagined that pain relief was something that had to be injected or inhaled, but one of the unexpected joys of home birth is that the home itself becomes a major source of comfort. Creating and honouring your partner's birth space is one of the most powerful ways that you can participate in this event.

James' Story
A yurt birth

James and his partner decided to create the ultimate birth space at their cliff-top home in New Zealand: a birth pool covered by a five-metre yurt (a kind of wood-framed tent used by Mongolian nomads).

The night before I put up the yurt, Kim had come back from the cinema reporting contractions every seven minutes. That got my adrenaline pumping. It was a night of checking the clock but, by morning, things had become quiet again. After breakfast I went to work and put up the wall and the door frame. As I was putting the rafters in place, I heard a loud splash in the ocean directly below. I turned to see the white wake left by . . . dolphins! There were about 20 bottlenose dolphins cavorting close to the base of the cliff, framed by the door of the yurt. If our baby landed there, or in the house, or in a hospital, I trusted that all would be well, but the possibility of her arriving here on this cliff top appealed to our romantic nature.

Kim's waters broke at 10pm, contractions started at 11pm, and we were in the birthing pool at around midnight. It was an ordeal for Kim (and for me as the support person) of eight hours of intense contractions, almost without break.

I retreated from the yurt to the house for a few minutes around 6am, leaving Kim in the very capable and gentle hands of our midwife. . . I could hardly contain my emotions; it was so hard watching my lover go through such pain, and I took a moment to break down and let my own tears flow. Once outside again, I looked at the stars for a few minutes, and then Kim's crying called me back.

When the moment finally came, it all happened very quickly. We had been out of the pool for about three hours, when Kim felt it might be helpful to go back in. At 6:50am, the baby's hairy head pushed through and, on the next push, it was all over. She came straight up onto Kim's chest to be embraced by us both and she gave a few little whimpers, but looked straight at us with big inquisitive eyes. She held her head up and looked strong and serene.

A perfect baby was born in a candle-lit yurt on a cliff top, in a birthing pool just as the sun came up!

Can my attitude during the birth influence my partner's perception of pain?

One of the most powerful tools for pain relief is already very familiar to you – in fact, it *is* you. Your attitude and actions during labour can make all the difference to your partner. As we've discussed in the first chapter, an anxious father can spread tension in the birth space, while a relaxed and confident father can provide his partner with the encouragement she needs to get on with the work of childbirth.

Different men have different ways of helping their partners to stay comfortable and calm during labour. Several of the fathers who contributed to this book suggested that 'keeping busy' was the best way for them to channel their fears into positive activity without causing their partner undue distress:

> ***If you start showing lots of fear, then everyone else will feed off it too. If you're going to freak out, just go out of the room and freak out for a minute and come back in again. I just tried to keep myself as busy as possible so I didn't actually sit down and go, Oh Jesus! (Bob)***

Other fathers cast themselves in more of an 'obedient servant' role, emphasising the importance of surrendering themselves to their partner's whims during childbirth:

> ***Do whatever they ask you for. Massage, massage, massage. Have all of the details worked out ahead of time, so that she doesn't have to even think about what needs to be done. (Jorge)***

For Bob, Jorge, and others like them, being 'useful' in whatever way the moment demanded was the best way that they could contribute to their partners' comfort.

Some men have identified a role of that went beyond practicalities and embraces a deeper sense of intimate support. Hannu from Finland remembers helping his wife through her most challenging moments, and he describes his labour support strategy as 'stay close – give space.' This approach may seem paradoxical – how can you stay close to your partner while also giving her space? But it describes a form of support that is nurturing without being overbearing. The man who stays close while giving space is not trying to 'fix' the problem of labour, nor is he intent on 'coaching' his partner through every contraction. He bears witness to her pain, letting her know that he is there when she needs him, retreating into a more passive role when she does not. 'Men like this often play a positive role,' suggests French obstetrician and author Michel Odent. 'They keep themselves in the background, sometimes even outside the room, as if to protect the privacy of their childbearing wives from the world outside.'[4] The idea of the man as guardian of the birth space becomes all the more pertinent during a home birth, when the space *is your* space, and you control who comes in and who goes out. By protecting the birth space, you give your partner the privacy she needs in order to retreat into the space within herself where labour can happen.

What about relaxation techniques such as hypnosis for childbirth?

The fathers in films and TV dramas often seem to give a non-stop colour commentary of their partners' labours. Adrenaline pumping, eyes fixed intently on the nether regions of their partners' hospital gowns, they repeat an endless mantra, 'Push, push, OK, now breathe, breeeeeathe, that's good, now pant, now breathe, you're doing great, honey!' While it's certainly possible that some women enjoy such coaching, it's more likely that a woman will respond to that kind of urgent instruction with a sharp glance, some blue language, or worse. Most women know instinctively when to breathe and when to push. Rather than attempting to tell your partner how to labour, it may be far more useful (and more enjoyable for both of you) to practice a gentler kind of communication.

In recent years, more and more couples have abandoned the kind of father-led coaching that became popular in the 1970s in favour of relaxation techniques that can be practiced during pregnancy and used throughout the various stages of childbirth. These techniques often involve the father (or doula, friend ,or other partner) guiding the birthing woman through a series of creative visualizations. For example, the woman might imagine her body opening up to labour and her baby's head moving easily through her pelvis; she might practice relaxing different parts of her body until all tension is released; or her partner might help her to recall the sights, sounds and smells of a special place where she felt calm and safe.

There are a number of CDs and books on the market that couples can use to learn and practice various 'scripts' for relaxation. If this technique appeals to you and your partner, you might choose to make these relaxation sessions part of your nightly routine during the later stages of pregnancy. Find a quiet time when you are unlikely to be interrupted by phone calls or older children, go to a comfortable place in your house, and guide your partner through a visualisation that she enjoys. Of course, your partner can do this on her own if she prefers. However, if she welcomes your involvement, then practicing these exercises together well in advance of her due date may help her slip into a state of deep relaxation more quickly and easily when the big day arrives.

Some couples who find these relaxation techniques effective and who enjoy working together as a birthing team go as far as to enroll in a series of hypnotherapy sessions before the birth. During these sessions, a father will not learn to put his partner in a trance and make her squawk like a chicken through her contractions. Instead, he will learn how to help her achieve a state of deep relaxation through the use of various scripts, massages and breathing techniques. Some practitioners of hypnosis for childbirth suggest that their methods can help women achieve completely pain-free labours, and research supports the notion that hypnosis offers most women at least a degree of effective pain relief.[5] Here, John from Scotland comments on his experience of learning and using HypnoBirthing, a popular brand of classes that teach hypnosis for childbirth:

> ***Jenni got [the hypnotherapist] to come out and have a chat with us and then we booked a HypnoBirthing course. We had six sessions, and they were very much about maintaining a sense of calm, and maintaining breathing. We did quite a lot of practice. The HypnoBirthing was great and definitely helped prepare us. I didn't know how long Jenni would be able to keep the breathing going for, but over 33 hours of labour, she did keep it going, just by maintaining focus and practicing what she was taught. (John)***

Some fathers find it difficult to learn the prescribed exercises and techniques of HypnoBirthing, not to mention keeping a straight face while doing so, but you need not necessarily buy a stack of CDs or a trimester's worth of classes to absorb the message that deep relaxation will help your partner to have a more comfortable labour. As Bob describes, in his pragmatic summary of the main message:

> ***Some of [the hypnosis methods] seemed extreme, because I thought, if she's going to be in the depths of agony, I'm not going to be able to pull her out of that by asking her to visualise a pink fluffy cloud. What did make sense was pulling out the important parts of the equation, like stress and fear equaling physical Tension, which equals your body not doing what it needs to do, which equals pain.***

You and your partner can find your own comfort levels with these techniques. Whether you're a 'pink fluffy cloud' man or not, relaxation and hypnosis are tools that are readily available and easily practiced before and during your baby's birth at home.

How should I touch my partner during labour?

It's free, it's easy, and it's something that you and your partner have practiced many times already: touch. Whether it's the squeeze of a hand, a warm embrace or a sensual massage, touch can often communicate your love more eloquently than words ever can. Massage, in particular, has long been a part of birth care in many indigenous cultures, and for good reason: gentle touch can be a reassuring counterpart to the overwhelming sensations that occur within a labouring woman's body, and touch can also be an effective way of communicating with a woman even after she withdraws into her internal 'labourland'. It is often difficult to give a labouring mother a massage in a typical hospital room, where she might have only a hard bed and a chair for support, and your hands might be impeded by a snarl of intravenous drips and wires. During a home birth, by contrast, your partner can assume whatever position she likes, wherever and whenever she wants.

If you and your partner often use massage as a way to relax or as part of your intimate time together, then extending this practice to the birth space will require little thought or adjustment. If, however, your attempts at massage are usually met with cries of 'Not there – there!' or 'Just forget it,' then you might be worried that you won't be up to the task on the day when it matters the most. Not to worry: some of the most effective massage techniques for labour are also the simplest. In the earlier stages of labour and during contractions, many women enjoy gentle massage of their shoulders and back or, perhaps, even a soothing foot rub. During contractions, you might try applying firm pressure to the sacral area of the lower back (the slight dimples on either side of your partner's spine, just at the top of her buttocks). You can press here or make slow circles with your thumbs, your fists or even your elbows. Some couples also use wooden or plastic massagers, and others have found that a tennis ball is a cheap and effective alternative that can be pressed or rolled over areas of tension.

You might choose to use a lotion or aromatic oil to make massage more comfortable for you and your partner; skin-on-skin friction can quickly become more of an annoyance than a comfort for all parties concerned. Anecdotal and clinical evidence suggests that, in addition to just 'smelling nice', essential oils can reduce anxiety, provide pain relief and even enhance the strength of uterine contractions when used during labour. In one study of over 8,000 mothers, oils of clary sage and chamomile were found to particularly effective,[6] although other oils such as lavender, geranium, jasmine, rose and neroli are also widely used for their relaxing and balancing qualities. These oils can be diluted in a base carrier oil, such as almond oil or wheatgerm oil, and they can be used for inhalation or hot compresses as well as massage. While you and your partner can buy many of these oils and experiment with different blends yourselves, an aromatherapist will be able to provide you with more advice about each oil's beneficial qualities.

So you've got your hands and you've got your oils – what next? Will you be doing a little massage for half an hour before wandering off to make coffee and sandwiches for your birth team, or could you be embarking on a massage marathon with no end in sight? Only time will tell. As Heath from New Zealand remarks:

> ***Maryanne required/requested lower back massage through every contraction from the moment I woke up to be with her, until our daughter was born 10 hours later.***

If you end up in a similar situation, bear in mind that massage can be effective even if you're not the one doing it. If you become exhausted (and if your partner is willing to give you a break), then another birth attendant, such as a doula, friend, or midwife, may be happy to take your place. Likewise, if your partner tells you 'Not there – there!' and swats your hand away for the umpteenth time, try not to take offense. It may be that your partner wants the intuitive touch of another woman. This is a normal response to the challenges of labour, and should not be taken as rejection of your loving efforts.

What about water birth? Is it safe? What are the benefits? And how do I deal with a birth pool?

Home birth allows your partner virtually unlimited access to another of nature's best pain relievers: water. You might imagine that water, like massage, is beneficial during birth simply because 'it just feels nice'. While the sensual pleasures of water are undeniable, research has also demonstrated that using a birth pool can accelerate labour, reduce a woman's need for drugs and surgical interventions, lower blood pressure, and reduce perineal tears.[7] The buoyancy and comfort of water also allow women to adopt more upright, gravity-efficient positions (such as all-fours or squatting) which might otherwise become tiring on dry land. Such positions are widely acknowledged to facilitate birth by encouraging the baby's swift descent and rotation. And, of course, water 'just feels nice.' Many a woman on the brink of desperation has sunk into her birth pool, only to sigh, moan, or even laugh as her immersion in warm water changed her contractions from miserable to manageable. The National Institute for Clinical Evidence (UK) suggested recently that all women should have the option of labouring in water. One of the consultant midwives who took participated in the study noted that water is 'the most effective form of pain relief barring an epidural in labour.'[8]

Your partner might achieve much-needed relief from a shower or a bath, but birth pools are often recommended as offering even greater benefit. Staying upright in a shower for hours on end can be exhausting, and changing positions in a bathtub may be difficult, if not impossible, for a labouring woman and her bump. Birth pools are large enough to allow more mobility, while still being providing an intimate, private space. In most areas, birth pools are available for hire or purchase in a range of styles. Some are inflatable, while others consist of fibreglass panels that must be bolted together. Most suppliers also offer a full range of accessories, including hoses, tap connectors, liners, covers, floating thermometers, and air and water pumps. If you do decide to use a birth pool, you and your partner might like to look at a number of different models before deciding which one best suits your needs.

For fathers, birth pools may sound dauntingly complicated – yet another logistical hassle to be overcome on the big day, when there are already so many things to worry about. Nonetheless, some men appear to relish the role of 'pool keeper'. Doing a few trial runs of filling and emptying the pool, preparing the pool on the day itself and keeping the water at an appropriate temperature helped many of the men who were interviewed for this book to focus their minds and gave to the experience a sense of purpose which might otherwise have been lacking. What's more, being in charge of something that provides your partner with such powerful pain relief can be gratifying for both of you, as Bob explains:

> ***My wife's always said that she would personally recommend the water as the best painkiller; the buoyancy of it took the weight off where she was uncomfortable, and allowed her to move around. One tip that the doula gave me was to pour water over her back during contractions – it was miraculous what that did for her. It was refreshing, and it helped to keep her in the room. She said the water was essentially the best painkiller she could have hoped for at the time.***

As labour progresses, you and your partner will probably find your own way of using the pool to maximum effect. Perhaps, like Bob's wife, your partner will also enjoy the soothing sensation of a stream of water over her back, perhaps she will prefer to lean back against the side of the pool with a warm towel draped over her belly, or maybe she'll ask you to massage her shoulders while she leans over the side. Maybe your partner will invite you to don your shorts and join her in the pool, or she might even suggest that you toss the shorts and scoot in beside her for a labour-day skinny dip. In the comfort and privacy of your own home, anything goes.

When it comes to your baby's arrival, your partner may feel more confident on dry land or she may choose to remain in the water. Research has shown that birth in water is safe for babies under the right conditions: the water must be kept at body temperature, in other words, at a temperature of about 37 degrees Celsius (98.6 degrees Fahrenheit), and the baby should not be handled or 'helped out' except for specific clinical reasons. In this way, the water in the pool will closely resemble the environment of the womb, and the baby's transition from one watery world to the next will be a smooth one. Moreover, the baby's 'dive reflex' will also prevent him or her from breathing while rising to the water's surface, and the umbilical cord will continue to provide a steady supply of oxygen. Many observers of water births have noted that this can be a wonderfully gentle way for a baby to enter the world. A midwife who is skilled and confident in water deliveries can help you to explore your options, and other couples who have welcomed their babies in this way may also be a rich source of information and inspiration.

Heath's Story
A watery labour

Heath is a purchasing manager from New Zealand who admits that he initially thought that home birth was 'something that tree-hugging people would do – a bit hippy-like!' Several months later, he found himself supporting his wife, Maryanne, at a joyful and straightforward home birth during which the birth pool served as one of the main sources of pain relief.

Labour began about 10pm, but Maryanne didn't wake me up until about 5am when the contractions were getting really strong, which was good because it meant that I was well rested to help her. When I woke, Maryanne needed me to rub her back through each contraction. We decided to phone the midwife at about 6am, and she came at 9am I felt excited that the day had come, and a little nervous with anticipation of a new beginning.

When the midwife arrived, we talked to her a bit and the atmosphere was very calm and peaceful. I continued to massage Maryanne's back through every contraction, and I started filling the birthing pool around 10am so that Maryanne could hop in for some pain relief. We were a bit nervous about doing this too early in case it slowed down the process, but the midwife checked Maryanne and found she was only two centimetres dilated, so we knew we still had some time to go. Maryanne got in the pool at around 11am; she was on all fours and I continued rubbing through the contractions. By this time, it was a very nice day outside, sunny, birds chirping outside the windows. A great day for our baby to arrive.*

As time went by, it seemed all of a sudden that Maryanne was about to give birth. Our midwife had called for the second midwife and she arrived within 10 minutes of Maryanne giving birth. I did notice her setting up things in the other bedroom (oxygen, towels etc) in case the baby needed assistance, but I wasn't really aware of what she was doing.

Maryanne got out of the pool with my assistance and knelt on our bedroom floor, leaning over the edge of the pool. The birth was under way. Maryanne was making a lot of noise, but she was doing really well with the assistance of the midwife. Because of the position Maryanne was in, I was very clearly

* Midwives often advise women not to get into the pool until labour is well established. Waiting until this time can help women take full advantage of the oxytocin surge that labouring in water can produce.

able to see the top of our baby's head during the pushing stage. It looked wrinkled and had very black hair. At this point it was very exciting, and I knew it wasn't going to be long before we had our baby to hold.

The pushing stage didn't seem to take too long. All of a sudden, there was a whole head. Maryanne rested for a small bit, and then all of a sudden a body and arms slipped out very quickly. As soon as the baby came out, I could see straight away that it was a girl. But I must admit I did leave it to the midwife to announce it to Maryanne, just in case I was wrong. The midwife held the baby as Maryanne turned around, we clamped the cord, I was able to cut it, and it was all very incredible. The placenta came out, but to be honest, I don't really remember much of that. Maryanne leaned back onto me as we sat on our bedroom floor, holding onto our little girl.

Maryanne went to have a shower, so during that time I lay on our bed with our little girl on my chest, all sticky & covered in vernix! By this time it was late afternoon, and the sun was setting outside our bedroom window. I remember feeling very warm, happy, and amazed.

Murray's Story

Born into water

Murray is a cardiac physiologist from Glasgow. He and his wife, Suzanne, chose a home water birth for their second child after the traumatic hospital birth of their first child, Keir.

The contractions must have started at about midnight. We called Suzanne's parents to come from their home an hour and a half away, and I phoned my parents to say that Suzanne was in labour. Then we called the midwives when the contractions were a certain space apart. Suzanne was doing breathing exercises, and the doula arrived shortly after we phoned her.

I went downstairs to get the pool up very quickly. I felt nervous, definitely, but also quite happy because we'd done the preparation and everything was ready. I knew how long the pool would take, and I was glad things had started at night because Keir was sleeping and we wouldn't have to leave him with anyone else that he didn't know. I felt a lot more comfortable that he was up there, and being in your own home, you know where everything is, you know your boundaries, you feel comfortable. Anyway, I set the pool up much more quickly than I'd done before – maybe it was the adrenaline! – and that was fine.

Suzanne came downstairs and she and the doula were doing breathing exercises. The midwives had arrived and they were telling us that everything was going well, they were doing their checks, and everything was just 'textbook'. Suzanne was coping really well with the pain and she was in and out of the pool; one position would be good, and then it would get sore after a while, so she'd move. The doula was coaching me as well, keeping me right, asking me how I was feeling, which was good – knowing that someone's taking an interest in how you're doing makes a big difference as well. It felt like a team effort when we were at home, as opposed to the hospital, where we didn't really have a clue what was going on.

The birth was amazing, really amazing. Suzanne was lying with her arms over the pool, and she was getting told to go with it, to push with the contractions. I looked down and the first thing I saw was a full head of hair underwater, jet black. Suzanne pushed again and his head came out and you could see his face, and then his arms came out and he started to make movements with his arms, and I remember saying, 'He's swimming, he's swimming!', and Suzanne was saying, 'He's still inside me!' The midwives were checking for the cord around his neck, and everyone was saying, 'That's great, you're doing really well', and one final push and he came out. He was swimming around in the pool underneath the water – it must have been five seconds but it seemed like forever – and it was just amazing.

Then the midwife picked him up, got him out the water, gave him to Suzanne, and they were both cuddling in the pool. We could see it was a boy and it was just amazing. Later, after they came out of the pool and went through to the 'nest' we'd made in the dining room, we had a moment to ourselves before Suzanne's parents came through. We had tea and coffee for the midwives and rounds of toast. It was good.

Can homeopathy provide effective pain relief at home?

Homeopathy is a system of complementary medicine that was developed by a German physician, Dr. Samuel Hahnemann, in the 19th century. Natural substances are diluted many times until a very small amount of the original substance remains, and this trace is then prepared in the form of tablets or powders. Before prescribing a treatment, a homeopath usually conducts an extensive 'interview' during which the patient's emotional, mental, and physical state are explored; a remedy that works for one person may not be advised for another with a similar condition.

Although homeopathy was once widely practiced and endorsed by many European doctors, it has become a favourite figure of fun for clinicians in recent years. In an era when medicine is increasingly standardised and less holistic, many doctors find it difficult to accept the notion that homeopathy works in different ways for different people at different times. Some doctors do accept that homeopathy may be beneficial, but they ascribe its benefits to the 'placebo effect' only. Newspapers regularly publish research in which homeopathy appears to have been disproved in the treatment of various conditions, while research that appears to support this alternative system often slips quietly under the mass media's radar.

The fact remains that many women – particularly those who plan to labour with minimal intervention – choose homeopathy to help them achieve a comfortable, healthy birth. Adela Stockton, a doula and homeopath, explains why this system of medicine may be so well suited to the time around pregnancy and birth:

> ***In contrast to the potential side effects and piecemeal treatment often attributed to orthodox medicine, homeopathy offers a safe and effective system of medicine that brings about harmony and healing within the human body as a whole. It is ideal for use during the childbirth year in that the remedies can support [a woman's] health at an emotional as well as a physical level . . .There may be times when [women] will benefit from the holistic rebalancing effects that homeopathy provides.***[9]

Just as birth is a continuum where a woman's emotional and physical states are seamlessly intertwined, so homeopathy claims to treat the 'whole self' without segregating mind from body. Many women choose to use homeopathic birth kits that contain a number of different remedies that are designed to meet the various emotional and physical challenges that birth can bring, from weak contractions to back pains to feelings of desperation, shock and weepiness. These kits can be purchased online and in some natural health shops, or they can be prepared to order by a local homeopath.

Understandably, a labouring woman may not be able to identify which remedies she requires at any given time, nor is she likely to remember to take these remedies at the prescribed intervals. These duties often fall to her birth partner, and if your partner would like to use homeopathy during birth, then you may well find yourself staring blankly at dozens of bottles of tiny white pills at four o'clock in the morning. It may be reassuring to know that homeopathic birth kits come with full instructions and recommendations, which can be studied before the birth, and you and your partner can discuss which remedies might be best suited to her when the big day comes. A recent study of women whose partners were trained in the administration of homeopathic birth kits noted that 'this had a positive impact on their birth partner's involvement.'[10] As with the use of relaxation techniques, massage, and a birth pool, you may find that improving your partner's emotional and physical wellbeing with homeopathy has gratifying benefits for you both. If, on the other hand, you are uncomfortable with the role of homeopathic helper and your partner still wishes to use this system of medicine, then these remedies can also be administered by another trusted birth attendant.

What are TENS machines, and how are they used?

Although home births are generally very natural, low-intervention affairs, it is still possible to labour at home while being hooked up to a machine – albeit a very small one. A TENS machine might look and sound like something out of a late-night science fiction film, but it is a popular choice for many home-birthing women. The machine consists of a small battery pack (about the size of an mp3 player) that sends electrical impulses along wires to four pads which can be placed on your partner's back – two just below bra-level, and two on either side of the base of her spine. Some TENS packs can be worn on a cord around a woman's neck or clipped to her clothing; all machines have settings that can be adjusted according to the strength of the contractions. A TENS machine set at a low level produces a light tingling sensation; a higher level feels more like a buzz. While your partner can change the setting herself from moment to moment, she may need some assistance to place the pads in the correct areas on her back.

You might be wondering whether a TENS machine's sole purpose is to provoke so much fumbling with wires, pads, and the like that the woman becomes momentarily distracted from her pain. While women often claim that putting on the TENS machine is, indeed, a welcome distraction in early labour, the machine is intended to work at a deeper level. TENS stands for

Transcutaneous Electrical Nerve Stimulation. In other words, this means that the machine's electrical impulses stimulate the body to produce its own pain-relieving endorphins, while also blocking pain signals from the uterus and the cervix to the brain. Clinical and anecdotal evidence appears to be divided on the effectiveness of TENS machines; some women find them uncomfortable or ineffective, while others swear by them. Women are advised to use TENS machines as early as possible during labour in order to build up a powerful cumulative effect, and some women do so, clutching their machine fiercely from the first twinge to the final contraction. Other women dislike the idea of using any kind of machine during labour, and would prefer to rely on lower back massage and/or water (neither of which can be used in conjunction with a TENS machine) for their primary pain relief. A TENS machine is another choice for your partner to explore and, apart from a bit of help with sticky pads and tangled wires, it is one which she can implement on her own.

What kinds of pain relief can the midwife provide at home?

Your midwife's most valuable tools are her heart and her hands. Her wisdom and sensitivity are paramount and, if she has chosen midwifery as a vocation rather than just an occupation, then she also brings with her a deep commitment to the natural birthing process. However, you may have noticed that, in addition to her heart, hands and good intentions, your midwife also brings an assortment of bags, boxes, crates and canisters to the birth. Most of the items in your midwife's kit are used to monitor and maintain the health of mother and baby but, in some countries, the midwife may also bring pharmacological pain relief in the form of Entonox and/or diamorphine.

Entonox (commonly referred to as 'gas and air') is a mixture of equal parts nitrous oxide and oxygen. It comes in large canisters and can be inhaled via a mouthpiece with a two-way valve. The labouring woman takes several deep breaths of Entonox as she feels a contraction building, then she eases off as the sensation reaches its peak and drifts away. Some women enjoy the feeling of giddiness or light-headedness that Entonox can produce, claiming that it 'takes the edge off' the pain, while others simply feel nauseous and perceive no major benefit. Although Entonox does enter a woman's bloodstream and cross the placenta, its advocates argue that the gas's high oxygen content is beneficial for the baby. Your partner may feel that the relief provided by Entonox is reason enough to use it. Alternatively, she may well try it and then abandon it, reassured that the gas will leave her system as quickly as it entered.

In some countries, midwives also have the option of bringing injectable opiates, such as diamorphine or pethidine, to home births. These substances have variable effects; some women find that opiates help them to relax and feel 'distant' from the pain, while others merely feel 'stoned', nauseous, or out of control. Diamorphine and pethidine can slow labour down and, because they cross the placenta, there is a possibility that the baby may be slow to breathe after birth and/or reluctant to feed.[11] Many women may be tempted to ask their midwife to bring these drugs in their birth kit, but they should be aware that such a request may open a Pandora's box. As Bob describes, having powerful drugs in the house can actually reduce a woman's confidence in her own ability to cope with pain:

> ***We had a long, drawn-out debate about how much pain relief to have in the house. The hospital would provide two canisters of gas and air, but then we came on to whether there should be anything else, meaning diamorphine or pethidine. The argument for it being, if we've got it there and the labour runs away from us and we lose control, then at least there's something there to have as back-up. But the other side was, if you know it's there, you're more likely to go, 'Oh, this is too hard, I'm taking an easy way out now.' If you know there are no drugs there, maybe you're more likely to stay focused. It's easy to say, 'Don't give it to me unless I'm begging and screaming for it,' but you don't know how it's going to go. (Bob)***

Anything that interrupts the natural hormonal sequence of birth needs serious consideration, especially if it might also have a negative effect on your child. However, these drugs are an option for many home-birthing women, and as such, your partner is entitled to make an informed choice about their possible introduction into the birth space.

No matter how your partner chooses to remain comfortable in labour, she can be confident that giving birth at home will allow her to explore her choices in her own way and in her own time. As for you, being in your own home will allow you to create and enhance your partner's birth space to her exact specifications, and to comfort her without fear of reproach from uninvited observers. In your own home, nobody can tell you that your music is too strange, your massage technique too haphazard, or your birth pool too large. With the right pain relief in place, you and your partner can ride the 'oxytocin wave' of labour in a way that a hospital environment would never allow.

5

Birth: Normal and Extraordinary

Prepare to be amazed. When the big day comes and only hours stand between you and your new baby's arrival, you and your partner will go on a journey through uncharted territory that is as awesome as it is challenging. This is the territory of birth, where each woman confronts and transcends her emotional, physical and spiritual limits. As an active participant in this process, you will also be tested – and rewarded – in ways you may not have imagined.

What can I expect a normal home birth to be like? What are the stages of labour?

Perhaps the greatest paradox of birth is that, although it is one of the most extraordinary events in human life, it is also one of the most normal. While every woman experiences birth in different ways, it is widely accepted that the birth process occurs in a series of distinct phases or 'stages'. There is no telling how long your partner will spend in any one of these stages, but knowing the rough sequence of events can be reassuring for both of you. Imagine you are both travelling through an unknown land: you do not know when you will reach your destination, which road to take, or how many false starts you will make before retracing your steps. However, you do know that you will pass at least a few definite signposts pointing you in the right direction. These signposts are the stages of normal birth and, regardless of how or when you see them, they will let you know that you and your partner are following the path to birth just as nature intended.

Early Labour

When does labour begin? There are as many answers to that question as there are women. The process of birth actually begins long before a woman's due date. From the very first weeks of pregnancy, her uterus begins to tone itself with regular, albeit imperceptible, contractions. As months pass and the baby's growth begins to stretch the uterus towards its maximum capacity, these contractions often become apparent as sensations of tightness or pressure. Many women find that these sensations can be triggered or intensified by fatigue, dehydration or physical activity, although this is not always the case.

In the days before any obvious signs of labour are present, the uterus continues to tone itself, and these Braxton-Hicks or 'practice' contractions may encourage the baby to engage or 'drop' into the pelvis. The baby's presenting part puts more direct pressure on the cervix, thus encouraging it to begin the process of effacement (thinning) and dilatation (opening).

While these remarkable physical changes occur, the last few days of pregnancy can also be emotionally intense. Some women experience the renowned 'nesting instinct', with sudden bursts of energy prompting them to tidy the house, tend the garden, or organise baby clothes. If you find your usually laid-back partner suddenly scrubbing the kitchen floor or trimming the front lawn with a pair of nail scissors, this could be a sign that things are about to happen.

For some women, early labour is a time of introspection, when many women who are normally active and gregarious find themselves instinctively staying closer to home and going about their day at a more peaceful, relaxed pace. As your partner contemplates the imminent arrival of your child, her feelings about this pregnancy and birth may be magnified. Her initial feelings about this baby – from doubt and fear to delight and joy – may resurface with renewed intensity.

As you and your partner explore and accept these emotions, early labour gives you both a chance to 'touch base' with each other one last time before the dynamic of your relationship shifts dramatically. You may be tempted to channel any nervousness into domestic chores – painting the baby's room, grappling with a new car seat, or doing a few more trial runs with your birth pool – but remember that this is also a good time to enjoy a few moments of stillness and intimacy. One of the most rewarding aspects of home birth is that early labour need not be a time of panic; your partner's first twinges won't have you dithering over the quickest route to hospital, or searching frantically under sofa cushions for loose change so that you can feed a parking meter in between stints in the labour suite. As a home-birthing father, you can relax and enjoy these last moments before labour begins in earnest. Whether you choose to give your partner a massage, share a special meal, go for a long walk, or spend a quiet evening with your older children, you can rest easy in the knowledge that you are already in the place where you need to be.

First Stage, or 'Active' Labour

Have you ever seen a woman go into labour on a TV sitcom or in a film? Did her waters break in a public place, with a loud and embarrassing gush? Did she then double over in pain, gripping a friend's hand with a white-knuckled fist, screaming desperately for an ambulance? While this scenario may be realistic for a very small fraction of the population, rest assured that most labours, particularly those of first-time mothers, have a much gentler and more gradual onset.

In the early phase of labour, your partner's 'twinges' escalate into more intense, regular, longer-lasting waves of pressure. At some point, it will no longer be possible for her to dismiss these feelings as mere backache or indigestion. Perhaps your partner's waters will break with a gush, perhaps they'll begin to leak with a slow trickle, or perhaps they won't break until your baby's head is actually crowning. Each one of these scenarios is normal and possible. Your partner may also experience what is sometimes euphemistically referred to as a 'show,' when the mucus plug that seals the cervix during pregnancy is discharged. The plug can resemble clear or pink-tinged jelly; it can come away all at once or in pieces. Excited by this unmistakable sign of labour, your partner may test the limits of your good humour by waving her soiled panty liner under your nose, or she may never notice the show at all. Again, either scenario is normal (even if the former comes as a bit of a shock to the system).

Some people claim that 'active' or 'established' labour begins when a woman's cervix has dilated to four centimetres. Your partner may or may not choose to call the midwife early in labour for an internal examination of her progress. Regardless of whether or not a midwife is present, it is likely that you will notice a distinct change in your partner's demeanour as labour intensifies. At some point, she may no longer be able to talk through her contractions; she may withdraw to that mythical place that is often referred to by midwives as 'Labourland', focusing her concentration entirely on these powerful surges. The noises she makes will change, she may feel restless, and she may ask you to draw near or to go away with little warning and for no apparent reason.

As her contractions become longer, more intense, and closer together, your partner will find her own personal rhythm and coping rituals. You may have lovingly prepared a 'labour playlist' of your partner's favourite music, but many women find comfort in listening to the same music over and over. Some women hum, moan, sigh or chant through their contractions; some laugh and some cry. All of these sounds are normal expressions of the intensity of birth. You and your other chosen attendant(s) can offer different kinds of support as your partner begins the birth journey in earnest. During active labour, some comfort measures lose their effectiveness, while others become lifelines.

Although the intensity of active labour may be overwhelming, you and your partner may still find moments of peace when you can 'check in' with each other and reflect on what's happening. Just as important is the need for you to 'check in' with yourself. If fear, panic or exhaustion threaten to overtake you, ask yourself why, and reassure yourself that this is OK. You may find it helpful to remind yourself that you are safe, your partner is safe, and your baby is safe. Staying attuned to your own feelings – and accepting them – will allow you to experience the fullness of the birth experience, and also, to provide your partner with more honest, meaningful support.

Transition

At some point, your partner's cervix will be fully dilated, that is to say, it will have reached a diameter of 10 centimetres, and will be wide enough for the baby to begin its passage down into the vagina. The next step is for your partner to push the baby out. However, before she can do this, she might experience a kind of intermediate stage known as 'transition'. During transition, contractions may appear to be relentless; they may last anywhere from 90 seconds to several minutes, with several peaks in each contraction and barely a break from one surge to the next. Even women who have coped well with labour up to this point can find this stage overwhelming. Many woman may appear panicky, desperate, or exhausted at this time, and it's not unusual to hear cries of 'Make it stop!', 'I'm going to die,' or 'I want to go home' – even during a home birth.

Transition is usually mercifully short compared to the active phase of labour that precedes it. However, it is a time when your partner is in particular need of constant support and affirmation. You can remind her that she's doing brilliantly, that she is strong, that she is beautiful, and that she will not die or break. It may be useful for both of you to remember that, although labour may seem impossible at this point, the physical and emotional intensity of transition are signs that birth is imminent.

Rest and Be Thankful

In 1753, soldiers inscribed the words 'Rest and be thankful' on a stone by the side of a notoriously treacherous road in the Scottish Highlands. This road, used by cattle drovers for hundreds of years, winds out of a deep and rugged glen and climbs to a staggering height before descending onto gentler terrain on the western edge of Loch Fyne. Although the road is now paved and somewhat less dangerous than the original rain-sodden path, the soldiers' words still serve as a timely reminder to travellers who have reached the highest point of this route.

You may be wondering what a wet Scottish road has to do with birth, but many women (in particular, first-time mothers) experience a lull in their labour after the intensity of transition, and this quiet phase is often given the name 'Rest and be thankful'. At this point, the woman has scaled the highest peaks of her birth journey; her contractions have built to a dizzying peak; and then, just before she enters the final stages of her baby's birth, things appear to slow down or, even, to stop altogether. It might be tempting to think that something is wrong at this point – how can the woman who was roaring like a lioness just a few minutes ago now be joking with the midwife and asking for a round of toast? The fact is that this stage may be nature's way of allowing women and their babies a chance to rest and recuperate before the final 'push' – both literally and metaphorically speaking – of labour.

The 'Rest and be thankful' stage can last anywhere from a few minutes to a few hours. A good midwife will be vigilant yet patient during this time; she can assess the vital signs of mother and baby at the usual intervals; and, if all remains well, then there is every reason to believe that labour will resume in due course. In the meantime, you and your partner should enjoy the break that nature has given you. By all means, rest, laugh, have a snack, go to the bathroom. Your baby will arrive when the time is right.

Second Stage

Remember that woman on television with her gushing waters, clenched fists and panicked cries? Let's revisit her, now, a few hours later. Here she is, lying back in a hospital bed, swathed in crisp sheets and surrounded by a tangle of wires and drips. Her feet are up in stirrups and, in between her thighs, here is the doctor, fully gowned, masked, scrubbed, and ready to catch the baby when it hurtles forth. The woman's husband is by her side; she holds his hand and looks searchingly into his eyes. 'Hold your breath!' he says, dutifully recalling the commands he's seen other men give their wives on other television shows. 'Put your chin down on your chest, keep holding that breath, and now, PUSH! Keep pushing! Keep it going, honey! You're doing great.' The woman does as she's told, her face contorting in a purple grimace, pushing for all she's worth until her husband finally says, '. . . aaaand relax.'

This kind of directed pushing is known as the Valsalva manoeuvre and, in many hospitals, it is still accepted as the standard way of 'managing' the second, or expulsive, stage of a woman's labour. However, most women feel their own urge to bear down once the cervix is fully dilated, and clinical evidence now supports the hypothesis that this kind of spontaneous pushing produces better outcomes for women and their babies than Valsalva pushing.[1] What's more, encouraging a woman to push whenever she wants, for as long as she wants, shows her that you believe in her ability to birth this baby in the way that only she knows best. Telling her when and how to push only undermines her intuition at a time when she most needs the support of those around her. At this time, you may want to encourage your partner to find the position that allows her to push most comfortably and effectively, such as standing, squatting, or kneeling on all fours. She may choose to breathe or sigh gently through each push, or she may roar loudly enough to be heard in the next town. You can support her as she seeks out the most natural and empowering way to bring your baby into the world.

During the second stage, many a father has been stymied by the sight of the top of his baby's head becoming visible, and then appearing to recede back into the vagina. This disconcerting phenomenon is normal and does not mean that your partner is doing things wrong. Although the baby may slip back slightly after each push, subsequent pushes should eventually result in the birth of your child. For some women, this pushing stage lasts just a few minutes; for others, it lasts a few hours. Once again, as long as your partner is well, the baby's heartbeat is healthy, and some progress continues to be made, then there is no need to rush. You can help by ensuring that the birth space remains warm, private and peaceful while your partner follows her most primitive impulses.

As your partner gives one last push and your baby enters the world, you may feel a rush of emotion. Many fathers describe this moment as 'amazing', 'incredible', 'unforgettable', or 'awesome'. A gush of waters or a wayward stream of baby pee can even lend a comical tone to the proceedings. No matter whether you laugh or cry, there is no doubt that this is a moment that you and your partner will remember forever.

Third Stage

In the months leading up to the birth, the focus is often so exclusively on the baby that it is easy to forget that birth doesn't end when the baby comes out. In addition to delivering your son or daughter, your partner must also expel the organ that has supported the child from the earliest moments of his or her existence: the placenta. From the Latin word for 'cake', your baby's placenta may not have swirly icing and trick candles on the top, but it is far more nourishing than most birthday confections. Lying against the uterine wall, the placenta transmits oxygen and nutrients to the baby via the umbilical cord. Birth is not complete until this amazing organ has been delivered, the umbilical cord has been cut, and your baby finally becomes a separate human being in his or her own right.

In a normal, physiological third stage, clamping and cutting of the cord are not urgent affairs. Parents who favour this approach generally choose to wait until after the cord has stopped pulsating. This delay has been found to allow the transmission of the maximum amount of oxygen and nourishment from mother to baby, providing benefits that last well into infancy.[2] While most parents who prefer such a physiological third stage are happy to cut the cord after a few minutes have passed and pulsation has stopped completely, some parents plan what is known as a 'lotus birth', during which the umbilical cord remains intact and the placenta is cleaned, dried, and kept close to the baby for several days until the cord dries up and breaks on its own.

Your partner can put the baby to her breast as soon as she wishes, and this interaction stimulates the release of the placenta. As the baby nuzzles into his mother's already familiar smell and drinks in the sweetness of his first feed, hormonal signals encourage the uterus to begin contracting once again. After some time – anywhere from a few minutes to several hours – the woman may feel a sense of heaviness and/or pressure and, after a few pushes, the placenta is born. This process should not be as painful or intense as the birth of the baby; after all, a placenta is boneless! In fact, many women experience feelings of exquisite release during the third stage. The work of birth is complete. For the first time since the beginning of the childbearing year, the womb is empty.

After the placenta has emerged, the midwife will check it to ensure that its membrane is intact, its lobes are healthy and complete, and no tissue has been left inside the uterus. Away from the protocols of the hospital and the eyes of strangers, you may have the chance to take your own sneaky peek at the placenta, if you wish. While nothing could be more stomach-churning for some men, others are intrigued by this organ whose vessels are often said to resemble a richly branched tree.

It should be noted that there is an alternative to a normal, physiological third stage, namely, an 'actively managed' third stage. Active management means that an oxytocic drug is injected into the mother's thigh just as her baby is being born. This drug encourages the uterus to contract strongly and the placenta to peel away from the wall of the womb. The umbilical cord is quickly clamped and cut, and the midwife may pull on the remaining cord to ensure that placental separation occurs. This practice was initially found to prevent postpartum haemorrhage in vulnerable women, and has since been routinely adopted as a preventative measure for most women in hospitals around the world. The advantage of this kind of third stage is that it is over quickly, in contrast to a natural third stage that may sometimes be a longer and altogether less predictable affair. However, some women find that the oxytocic drug used in an actively managed third stage makes them feel nauseous or faint, and the cord pulling or 'traction' that follows can be uncomfortable if it is performed by a less-than-gentle attendant. Because the oxytocic injection encourages the uterine veins to constrict so aggressively, there is also an increased risk that some placental tissue may be retained in the uterus, and such remnants can cause severe infection if not removed. From a more philosophical perspective, you and your partner may simply be wary of any intervention that interrupts the natural sequence of hormones in the first few crucial moments after birth. As such, it might be wise to research your third-stage choices well in advance of the birth itself.

Regardless of whether you and your partner choose a normal, physiological third stage or an actively managed third stage, you may be wondering what actually happens to the placenta after it comes out. The midwife usually offers to take the placenta away and dispose of it, either by incineration or by donation to medical research. However, you also have the choice of keeping the placenta for yourselves. In many indigenous cultures around the world, the placenta is seen as part of the child, and to dispose of it or send it away would be a gross breach of the baby's dignity. Parents who honour the placenta's symbolic significance may choose to bury the placenta in their garden, sometimes planting a tree above it, as this woman describes:

In New Zealand (Aoterearoa), Maori have a name for belonging to a place: they call it their Turangawaiwai, which is also their name for the placenta. It is an increasingly common practise for many New Zealanders of all ethnic origins to take the placenta home and plant a tree over it. Our children really appreciate it. 29 years on, my daughter knows where she belongs: under the walnut tree in Nanna's garden.[3]

If you and your partner choose to bury the placenta, you may need to make sure that you do so in accordance with local environmental health policies, a process which, as George describes below, is not without its own logistical challenges:

Leanne regretted that the midwives took the placenta and didn't leave it with us. They told us we'd need to bury it in a hole six feet down, and I thought, 'No way, that's too much!' Although now, of course, we've heard stories that nobody digs that deep. So maybe we should have kept it to put in our garden without excavating six feet.

Policies related to burial of placentas can vary from region to region, so it might be worth checking with your own local authority well in advance of your home birth.

In addition to believing in the placenta's spiritual significance, some parents also believe that the organ has powerful medicinal qualities. American movie star Tom Cruise raised eyebrows in 2006 when he indicated that he and his fiancée would eat the placenta after the birth of their first child, but this practice of 'placentophagy' is much more than just a Hollywood fad. Advocates point to the fact that most mammals eat their own placentas after birth and they suggest that women who do so may be replenishing their iron stores and ingesting hormones that might help to stave off postnatal depression. If your partner likes the idea and fancies a bite of placenta to perk her up, then recipes for roasted, stewed and casseroled placenta abound on the Internet. If, however, neither of you can stomach the idea of a placenta lingering in your freezer, simmering on your stove or sizzling on your plate, then there is always the more conventional and, some might argue, just as uplifting option of a cup of tea and a generous slice of chocolate cake.

The stories that follow illustrate the vast spectrum of normal birth better than any clinical descriptions ever could. As you read them, you will see that some labours are long, some are short; some women delight in their contractions while others struggle against them; and some fathers play a central role in the birth process while others prefer to watch from the sidelines. However, the births that are described all have one thing in common: they are all 'normal', in spite of the differences and variations. Let the wisdom and humour of these fathers reassure, inspire and entertain you as you and your partner work towards your own home birth choices.

Duncan's Story
A home birth convert

At first, New Zealander Duncan was extremely skeptical about the idea of a home birth. However, after the safe arrival of his son, Duncan's attitude has changed from cynical to evangelical.

It all started for me some three and a half years ago at an antenatal class for expectant, first-time parents, sitting with a group of strangers, wondering what the hell I was doing there. Midwives! Bring on the doctors, the machinery, the drugs, and the other wonders of modern science. But here I was, dragged along by my wife's excitement, listening to what I thought at the time was the 'hippy' section of the medical profession, subscribing to nature's way and homeopathic remedies for childbirth. These, I thought, were the people probably not good enough to get a job at the hospitals. How wrong

I was! In hindsight, women have been giving birth for quite a few years, and why I thought giving birth in a hospital would be better, I have no idea.

Now, onto the birthing part. I remember organising the birthing pool, which I wanted to collect from the hire place four months before the due date, just in case. Apparently, this is not allowed, and I ended up collecting it about three weeks before my son arrived. We were organised: birthing pool, seven hundred thousand square metres of heavy duty polythene (apparently there would be blood and stuff everywhere, or so I was told), and some old sheets. With bubbly, Camembert, and pâté in the fridge, we were ready to go.

The big day: Ange awoke on the due date and had some crampy things. (I've never really understood what that's all about, but I have sympathised with her all our married life.) Anyway, she had had these before, so no real panic at this point. We just carried on with breakfast and the other normal things people do on the weekends.

Another hour or so, and the cramps were a little worse and the toilet was continually occupied – not a great day to relax and read the weekend Herald. Perhaps this was it. Having not been there before, I was unable to offer any pearls of wisdom as to whether or not labour had started, but it had.

Lunchtime came, things were a little more serious and it was time to ring the midwife, who arrived not long after with the usual spiel that if you're not sure you are in labour, then you're probably not. Midwives are not perfect – we were in labour. (You will notice that I use 'we', as it was difficult for me to watch my wife in pain, and as a man who wants to fix things, it was difficult not to be able to do anything about it other than let nature take its course.) The midwife explained that we were only four centimetres dilated and that, as a rule of thumb, we could expect one centimetre per hour, so still six hours to go. She left (with our permission) to go and call on a couple of other clients and we were left to it.

Anyway, time for 'Action Man' – polythene spread out to cover the entire lounge, the furniture, and half way up the walls (I was planning for a war zone!). Towels and old sheets were spread out, the pool up, and filling commenced. Let me tell you, those pools are big. No trouble with the cold water, but the hot water cylinder was drained, so I had pots out and boiling on the stove along with the jug and anything else that I could find to fill up that pool.

Things were starting to get more intense, with Ange unable to get comfortable: stand up, sit down, lie down, stand up, walk around. All the while, I was not quite sure what she wanted me to do, so I hovered, getting cold flannels, rubbing her back, bringing cold drinks, etc., just to be there for whatever she wanted. I thought I did a pretty good job, but you probably need to check with her to see if I did the right things or not. Big thing here is, just do whatever they want, and life will be perfect.

I phoned the midwives when Ange felt like she needed to push, and they arrived about 30 to 40 minutes before Lucas turned up in the pool, to the absolute delight of his father.

Guys, I consider myself to be pretty much a man's man, but let me tell you: nothing prepares you for the sheer overwhelming joy and love you feel when your child is born. Also I had some dust in my eyes which made my eyes water. (My wife will try and tell you that I cried, but that simply is not true.)

I am not going to try and tell you whether you should have your baby at home, in a hospital, or at a birth centre – that's your decision. What I will say is that for me, having my son at home has been the best decision we ever made, despite my initial concerns. To be able to spend that time with my wife pretty much on our own was just such a tremendous privilege; no doctors, no smell of disinfectant, no machines beeping. Just the comfortable feeling you have when you sit at the place you live in. You know where everything is and visiting hours never end. There was no rush to cut the cord, no rush to do anything, and best of all, I got to be the first person to dress my son and pass him onto the most amazing woman I know: my wife.

Mika's Story

'I can't believe it!'

Mika is a research engineer from Finland who was initially unconvinced by his wife's enthusiasm for home birth. Their first son's hospital birth had been traumatic, and both Mika and his wife were worried that history might repeat itself. However, as the following story shows, home birth turned out to be much more straightforward than Mika or his wife had expected.

My wife was two weeks overdue and we were ready to go to the hospital soon for an induction. It was Friday morning and Milla felt some rushes, some of which stopped her from standing or walking. She called our midwife, who told us to keep calm. However, things were developing quite quickly, so I started filling up the birth pool and we called our midwife again so that she would come.

We waited for our midwife and there was very little going on. My wife concentrated on her labour and I finished filling the birth pool and made some breakfast for our son. Everything was going well. I started timing the rushes, just to have something to do. Sometimes during the peak of a rush, my wife was quite loud, but that didn't seem to bother our son. I myself had made up an attitude to wait for worse. We lived in an apartment building, so I put a note on our door saying something like, 'We are having a home birth. Sorry for the possible disturbance. We have a midwife, no other help needed. Thank you!'

When the midwife arrived, I then had something to do, as she needed some space for her equipment and she asked for a few different things. And then I could see her examining Milla and asking her some questions. Our midwife was a very calm person and she knew Milla didn't like too much interference, so she mostly observed the situation and just let us know that everything was going well.

I mostly played with our son, who was taking everything very well. I got some clothes for him so that if he felt uncomfortable, we could go outside. Our apartment had only two rooms and the birth pool was in the middle of our living room, so being inside meant being in the middle of the labour, but it really didn't seem to bother him – he was still able to eat and play. I took some photos and we really just waited for something to happen. My wife isolated herself from everything and didn't seem to like it when the midwife tried to examine her or even touch her to ease the pain.

*Then, quite suddenly, the midwife said that she saw the baby's head. I was surprised because there had been no signs that we were so far already, and my wife seemed to be very surprised herself. Then things happened very quickly. The midwife told my wife to stand up, because the water was green.** *This was the time we were a bit afraid, I think. Our first son had been helped out with a suction pad and his birth had really been quite difficult – it had felt like it was never-ending, waiting for the pushing and the immense*

* *Author's note:* Amniotic fluids or 'waters' are usually clear or slightly straw-coloured, but when fluid is green, it is usually a clear sign that the baby has had a bowel movement while still inside the womb. This is sometimes – but not always – a sign of fetal distress.

pain to be over. This time, though, everything was over before we even realised. The baby popped out without much effort. My wife just repeated 'I can't believe it', probably meaning that she had been waiting for much more work and pain.

I needed to help the midwife right away because she had to untie the umbilical cord, which was wrapped around the baby. We helped my wife out of the pool, the midwife quickly had a look at the baby to check if she was okay, and to let us know that she was a girl. Then she gave her to my wife. We were just very happy and I helped our son to have a look at his new little sister. The midwife stayed with us for a while to see that everything was good, but everything went back to normal pretty quickly. For my wife, it was clearly very important to be in a familiar environment right after the birth – she was very, very happy.

Bob's Story
Born in the nick of time

Bob is an artist from Scotland. He and his wife, Bec, chose to have their first baby at home in spite of opposition and incredulity of friends, family, and medical staff. Bec's hopes for a home birth seemed futile when she went past her due date and a scan revealed a potentially alarming low level of amniotic fluid, but on the day before she was scheduled for induction, her labour began.

I'm not sure what did the trick, be it the extra spicy curry, the tinned pineapple, the long walks, the bouncing, or the raspberry leaf tea, but I suspect the mere threat of induction was probably the trigger. Bec woke me in the wee hours of Friday to tell me she was having some cramping. Now, see, at the antenatal classes, they always said that you will know, without hesitation, when you are in labour, but we were both so anxious about our deadline that it felt impossible to know how to react to the slightest change. Some phone calls to the hospital and an hour later we went back to sleep – there was nothing to worry about yet, it seemed.

However, the cramps didn't disappear that day, and Bec did appear markedly more uncomfortable as we wheeled the trolley around the supermarket on our weekly shop. We returned home and called the hospital and Leah, our doula for advice. Again, it seemed there wasn't too much to get our hopes up about, but nonetheless, a midwife would be dispatched just to give Bec a wee once-over. I can confirm that since then, I do get a little nervous flush whenever I walk into the supermarket.

Leah arrived shortly and agreed that Bec may indeed be in the early stages of labour. She also helped attach our rented TENS machine. The midwife arrived a little later and did an examination to determine just exactly where we were up to. To everyone's surprise, or total jaw-drop, Bec was already more than half way there. The back-up midwife was sent for.

As it turned out, the TENS machine had a loose connection and had to be abandoned. Leah had provided us with a birthing pool, which became Bec's only source of pain relief. Throughout labour, the first midwife and her back-up provided a very discreet monitoring of the baby's heart, but otherwise they kept to the sidelines with their cups of tea. Leah massaged Bec and complemented this with some aromatherapy, whilst I generally tried to cheerlead as best I could and kept the refreshments coming. Bec was amazing as she quietly breathed her way through it in complete control. As a Sigur Rós album serenaded us in the candlelight, Bec turned herself over to the birthing process in the pool and, only seven hours after our team had been assembled, we were in the final throes. A hasty position swap at the last moment allowed me the beautiful experience of catching Casper as he was delivered and telling Bec the sex. Casper spewed all over me in mid-air as he flew into my arms, and then promptly pooed all over his mummy as I handed him up to her, ensuring that the love was spread around nicely for both of us. I cut the cord, or at least attempted to – the blunt scissors I was handed for the task made the experience akin to carving a steak with a teaspoon – but eventually we got there and baby stepped (well, tumbled) into the world as his own man.

Rajiv's Stories

Two home births, short and sweet

It is often the mother-to-be who introduces her partner to the idea of home birth, but in Rajiv and Anne's case, the roles were reversed. Having grown up in France, where medicalised birth is the norm, Anne was wary of the idea. Although Rajiv was born in a hospital in Scotland, the home births of his three sisters in India gave him confidence in the safety and normality of home birth from an early age. The couple's first child was born in London, as Rajiv describes here.

What happened with the first birth was, we'd got some of my family and Anne's family over for dinner at around 8pm. Anne realised things were happening because she had a show, so we finished dinner by nine or ten and then we had to get rid of our guests. Anne's brother and my sister-in-law were a bit puzzled as to why they were being asked to go.

Anne started to pace around and try to get comfortable as the labour started. I was feeling quite excited and nervous because, if the show was there, chances were that something was going to happen soon, but I didn't want to get over-excited because we were both expecting the labour to be long-ish. It was all fairly calm at the beginning; we turned all the lights off.

Anne wandered around and was quite agitated by trying to manage the contractions. They weren't regular, but they were quite strong, not like how you see in movies – that's all bullshit! Some of the things you see in movies, it's like, love doesn't happen that way, so why should birth? Anyway, Anne walked around and became more and more agitated. I was trying to measure the contractions because, this being our first baby, we thought that would be important. By agitated, I don't mean in a bad sense, I just mean she was really starting to feel the pain and regretting her choice about medication at that point. She thought the pain was going to last for ages and ages and she wouldn't be able to handle it but, in fact, she was about to give birth.

I called the midwife again, and this time she thought she really ought to come over, so she threw her clothes on over her pyjamas and was there in about 15 or 20 minutes. By the time she arrived, even I could see that the baby was crowning, and the midwife had just enough time to phone the second midwife and ask her to come quick. Anne found a position that was comfortable, and when my daughter's head popped out, it was just the most amazing thing in the world, absolutely amazing. I was thinking, 'Oh my God!' Anne held the baby to begin with, but then I held the baby just when Anne went to get cleaned up, and it was absolutely wonderful. It is messy, the baby's covered with vernix, but it doesn't matter at all. The mess is completely irrelevant – don't be afraid of it.

It was a tremendous experience. There we were at home: Anne was having toast and hot chocolate and feeding the baby, and I was making phone calls, and this was all happening by six in the morning.

By the time Rajiv and Anne had moved to Glasgow several years later and conceived their second child, they didn't hesitate to plan another home birth.

With the second birth, we were more aware of what was going to happen, and it was easier for us because we knew what to expect. When labour started, we relaxed into it more, we felt a bit less fearful. We didn't expect the contractions to be regular; Anne had a better sense of when things were going to happen.

Anne got into the bath this time, which really helped a lot with the pain. Then we just organised the bathroom; there was a big bath, soft lighting, and it really worked well for us. The only thing I really remember was that the bathroom filled with steam and it was tremendously hot, we were sweating away, but a warm room is good for the baby, so that's fine. Because this baby was born underwater, I could see the head pop out in the water – a head of hair, which is what you'd expect with Indian babies – and then he was born within a minute or two. It was really wonderful. It was a bit less traumatic for us this time because it was more like what we were expecting.

Both births just felt incredibly calm afterwards. You get on with cleaning up or whatever, although with the one in the bath, there was very little to clean at all, just a few towels. The sense of calm and relief afterwards . . . it really is a very happy time.

Scott's Story
No more sports cars

Scott's first child, Eimii, was born in a hospital in New Zealand. However, after moving to London and conceiving a second child, some pro-home-birth comments from a cricket teammate prompted Scott to raise the issue with his wife, Michelle. The rest, as they say, is history.

It was early Saturday morning and Michelle popped her head in the bedroom door at 8.30 to say that she thinks her waters have broken! My first task was to ask Michelle if she was sure, and once she had confirmed that she was pretty sure, I called the midwife to tell her that our baby was on the way.

The midwife wasn't in a particular hurry to come over because she thought she had another 30 hours ahead of her before the baby arrived. However, I had to tell her that our first child arrived after only five hours and 29 minutes and I thought child number two would arrive in a similar time too!

Both our daughter and I were really excited! After nine months of waiting, we were finally going to get our baby! In particular, the previous nine months had been agony for our daughter, as she had really struggled to contain the excitement of getting a new sister.

So the midwife and her student arrived about an hour and a half after I first called, and I went down to help them drag several tons of what looked like scuba air tanks into our house. What was really nice was how excited the student was! As this was her first home birth, she was taking all sorts of notes and being as helpful as possible. She really was quite excited about everything happening in front of her.

At 1.30pm, our baby finally made its grand entrance. The single thing that stands out the most is how the bump in the tummy goes down as baby is coming out! It's just not something you really think about until you have seen how rapidly that bump disappears when baby arrives.

During this time, our daughter, who had been standing by the door taking everything in, became quite fascinated and was getting in so she could see baby being delivered. Prior to that, whenever we mentioned the delivery of her sister, she had squirmed and shied away but, on the day itself, she was trying to take in as much as possible.

The emotions I felt as that small little baby was placed on my lovely wife's tummy are indescribable! The love, the relief, the joy was welling up inside me. Here was this small, little thing who was totally dependent on my wife and me, and she was all ours! We had tried for a number of years to have more children and earlier in 2006 we had decided to give up and buy a two-door sports car. However, just when all hope seemed to have gone, along came our little miracle...and now she was here!

The home birth, and how our family pulled together, was the culmination of three years of having to live in a foreign country, in a large unfriendly city, twelve thousand miles from the nearest family. That day has been a high point in our family life.

George's Story
A sunny day, an easy birth*

The hospital birth of George's first child was traumatic for his wife, Leanne: she was given limited choices during her labour, the postnatal ward seemed busy and chaotic, and there were three fire alarms on her first night with her new baby. Years later, when George and Leanne conceived their second child, home birth promised a calmer, more empowering experience. An economist by profession, George weighed the probabilities and decided that the odds were in favour of a healthy baby and a happy mother.

* Names in this story have been changed at the contributor's request.

It was a nice sunny day at the end of October, and Leanne felt that the labour might be starting, although very irregularly. We decided to speed it up a bit by taking a walk, and we have a nice walk near our home, on a nice path away from the road with a small river running by. So we all went for a walk: me, Leanne, our daughter, and my mother-in-law, who had been staying with us and helping out. After walking for about an hour, we came back, and the contractions became more regular.

We had our normal lunch and, at about four or five, Leanne called the midwives, and they said they were coming. I wasn't worried at all because this was our second child, and we had this gap of nine years – we had grown older, and maybe we had learned to take life easier. Looking at the positive side and having a nice sunny day, I didn't worry – not at all. From my point of view, I was in between jobs, so I had no obligations or demands on my time, I didn't need to rush anywhere or worry about waking up the next morning and going to work. I took it as it came – absolutely normally.

At around six o'clock in the evening, my daughter ran a hot bath for Leanne, so she had a relaxing bath, which you can't usually have in a hospital. I think it all started developing faster by about eight in the evening. Leanne didn't take any painkillers; she'd had an epidural the first time around, but either she was better prepared or relaxed more at home this time, or maybe it was easier, or maybe it was a little bit of everything together. My mother-in-law and I were helping Leanne, and our daughter helped a lot too, even though she was only nine – she gave Leanne a cold cloth to wipe the sweat off her face. The midwives were having tea and chatting over the newspapers in the kitchen; they weren't immediately necessary. It was all quite nice; we had a safe feeling and a good environment.

Then the baby was born, just . . . hup! Leanne was on her knees, leaning over the bed, and the baby was immediately given to her to hold. The cord was quite short, so then I cut it as I had done for our first baby. Then our daughter held him, and then he immediately started thinking about milk. I felt very satisfied.

The only problem was that the placenta hadn't come after two hours. Leanne didn't want to keep the midwives longer and maybe they didn't want to stay either, so they gave her an injection to get the placenta out faster. It worked, and it was the only thing that didn't go the natural way. I don't really worry about it, although Leanne may have a different opinion.

Tim's Story
An intimate experience

When Tim met his partner, Grace, she was already pregnant as the result of a prior relationship. The couple remained committed to each other, and Tim agreed to support Grace through pregnancy and birth. As he describes here, it was an emotionally charged experience, especially as Grace had already decided to give the baby up for adoption. This story illustrates the importance of 'checking in' with oneself and one's partner: exploring and accepting the full range of emotions that any birth can bring.

I woke up at about 10 o'clock in the morning. Grace had been up since about seven, and she said, 'It's started, I'm going to have a baby today.' And I thought, 'Great, brilliant!' That was quite terrifying, actually. So I got up and made lots of cups of tea, sorted out the house, tried to keep everything tidy, put down tarpaulins on the floor, got the pool pumped up, and turned on the heating. I went out and got a few mango smoothies and that sort of thing.

When I came back, Grace laboured on, and we sat with one another quite a lot. There was a lot of sexual contact as well that day, like we were in a little cocoon together, you know. Then we had a big, huge, spicy curry and some more raspberry leaf tea, and we went out for a proper big walk – a hard walk. It was lovely, actually. It was a nice day, quite sunny, and Grace had her shades on and was stopping every three minutes to go, 'Oooh!'

We came back, and maybe at about seven that night, we phoned Allison, the midwife, to come down. As soon as she came, things slowed down and started going off again, and I was just doing bits and pieces and holding Grace's hand in the dark, that sort of thing.

It must have been about one o'clock or two o'clock in the morning that it really started going, and it was quite obvious that something was going to happen. I called Allison. Grace was in the bedroom and Allison came in and was very, very hands-off and let the baby come out. It was dark, and I had to hold the torch so Allison could see what was going on, which seemed really an amazing thing to be doing at the time. The baby came out and I remember it being caught and the cord still being attached, and immediately Grace picked it up and started to breastfeed, and it was really perfect and meaningful; it was just instinct. Amazing.

At that point, I got really, really, really emotional, like a blubbering wreck, and I actually had to go out into the garden and leave those two together for a little while. The massive emotional impact had actually come after the birth, and obviously it was magnified because of the surrounding circumstances as well – the fact that we had to give the baby up. That might be the part that's quite difficult for men; certainly it was difficult for me, being so involved for nine months, and then immediately when the baby came out, feeling so detached from the situation. Maybe that was just me, but I found that quite difficult. It's not that I felt any jealousy at all, I just wasn't part of the process anymore, and rightly so: all of Grace's attention was on this child, and I didn't want to take any attention. I hadn't cried like that in years and years. It was very strange.

So then I came back in and the practical things started happening; the umbilical cord got cut and Grace had to go and do a few things. I held the baby for a while and had a really lovely time. Then the adoptive parents came round and we gave the baby over, and it was very, very bizarre – the strangest situation, really. Grace was far more put together than I was. I was completely wrecked, but it was still absolutely beautiful and an incredible experience to have, such an act of giving on Grace's part – unbelievable to see. During the whole birth, I really saw what Grace was capable of, and what women are capable of in general, and I either hadn't seen that, or hadn't allowed myself to see that before.

6

Challenges and Complications

While the majority of healthy women with straightforward pregnancies go on to have straightforward births, it would be foolish to suggest that complications never occur. Most challenges that arise during labour can be resolved without major clinical intervention. In some cases, patience is all that is needed. In others, the midwife's skill and resourcefulness may be more strenuously tested. A small proportion of cases may require transfer to your chosen birth centre or hospital, where the full array of modern technology is available if and when it is truly necessary.

By making the decision to birth at home, you and your partner have already demonstrated your faith in birth as a normal, healthy process. However, not even the most supportive father is immune from the 'what ifs'. These 'what ifs' can strike when you least expect them. For example, as you fill the birth pool, stock the fridge with your partner's favourite fruit juice, or share an intimate massage on the eve of labour, a small but persistent voice may interrupt your preparations: 'What if she can't cope with a long labour? What if the cord is around the baby's neck? What if we have to go to the hospital?' This voice doesn't mean that you're unbalanced; it simply means that you're human. Doubts and fears are normal at any stage, and if the doubts prompt you to become better informed about what lies ahead, then your fears might very well be calmed.

This chapter is not an encyclopedic guide to the quirks and variations of birth, but it will answer a few of the most common 'what ifs'. In addition, you will learn about some of the things you can do to help if events should take an unexpected turn. Many fathers worry about feeling helpless or useless during labour, and that worry can be amplified when things go wrong. However, there is almost always something you can do to support your partner even – and sometimes, especially – in the most challenging situations.

What if my partner goes into labour prematurely? Can we still have a home birth?

Premature or 'preterm' birth is often defined as birth that occurs before 37 weeks of pregnancy. Prior to 37 weeks, there may be a risk that the baby's lungs are not mature enough to allow him or her to breathe independently. If your partner has a history of miscarriage or preterm labour with previous children, then she may be at risk of having an early birth with this baby. Some midwives are happy to attend a home birth from 37 weeks onwards, while others will not attend until at least 38 weeks have passed. If your partner goes into labour well before that point, she will almost certainly be asked to come into the hospital, where she can be more closely monitored and your baby can receive special care immediately after birth. However, if labour begins at or just before 37 or 38 weeks and you wish to be attended by a midwife, your partner may well be able to achieve a home birth, depending on circumstances and your midwife's willingness to monitor and attend her as planned.

What can I do to help?

There is no magic wand you can wave to ensure that your baby emerges perfectly 'cooked' and ready to go at exactly 40 weeks of gestation. However, there are some strategies that you and your partner can discuss during her pregnancy. Research suggests that a healthy diet can be essential in optimising the chances of a full-term birth. In particular, one study noted that eating oily fish at least once a week (or taking fish oil supplements) can dramatically cut the risk of preterm delivery.[1] Numerous studies also indicate that stress can be a major factor in prematurity: science and common sense both suggest that a woman who feels safe and secure is more likely to have a healthy pregnancy and birth. If your partner appears overwhelmed by work commitments, housework, care of older children, or any other issues in the months leading up to the birth, then it may be helpful to discuss whether you can ease her load by offering emotional or practical support of any kind.

What if the baby is overdue? Can we still have a home birth, or should my partner be induced in the hospital?

In order to answer this particular 'what if', we first need to explore the definition of 'overdue'. Modern medicine has various ways of determining when your baby is actually 'due.' The most prevalent method for calculating an estimated date of delivery (EDD) is based on work done in 1850 by Dr. Franz Carl Naegele, a German doctor who deduced that most births occur an average of 266 days after conception. However, Dr. Naegele assumed that most women have a 28-day menstrual cycle and that they ovulate on exactly the fourteenth day. You may only have a passing familiarity with your partner's menstrual cycle but, if she is like millions of other women around the world, then chances are that her cycle hardly goes like clockwork. Since Dr. Naegele's time, research has indicated that the average duration of gestation is more like 280 days, but further analysis (and a wealth of anecdotal evidence) suggests that this figure can vary widely, depending on factors such as parity (whether a woman is having her first or subsequent birth), ethnicity, seasonal variations and work patterns.[2,3,4]

Naegele's system and its variations are not the only ways of determining due dates. The advent of ultrasound has given doctors another way of dating pregnancies. However, this technique is based on the assumption that all babies conform to a 'norm' of size and weight at certain stages, it becomes less accurate as the pregnancy progresses, and it is subject to human interpretation and error. Weight gain, hormone levels in the blood, fundal height (the distance from a woman's pubic bone to the top of her uterus) and the time of 'quickening' (when the baby's first movements are felt) are also potential, albeit imprecise, indicators of the stages of pregnancy. Even if you know exactly when your baby was conceived, there is no surefire way of knowing exactly when he or she will be ready to be born.

Your partner may be quite happy to go along with the EDD that she's been given, or she may regard the date with an attitude of distinct mistrust. Many a woman has been heard to tell her girlfriends, 'The doctor says I'm due on this date, but *I just know* my cycle was irregular / I conceived a week before they think I did / my babies are always early / all of the women in my family go two weeks overdue.' Some women who routinely have 'overdue' babies head off this conflict at the outset by telling their midwife or doctor that their last menstrual period arrived several days or a week later than it actually did, thereby assuring themselves of a later EDD. As with so many aspects of pregnancy and birth, a woman's intuition often turns out to be correct, when all is said and done.

It is, in fact, virtually impossible to say with certainty when a baby is actually 'due', or, for that matter, when the baby is dangerously 'overdue'. Your healthcare providers may or may not adhere rigidly to your partner's EDD, and depending on how flexible they are willing to be, your partner may or may not experience increasing pressure to have her labour induced as the hours and days tick by. Your partner may be lectured about the risks of going 'post-dates'. Indeed, many women are warned that their placenta will deteriorate or their amniotic fluid will reach dangerously low levels if they choose to remain pregnant after a certain amount of time has passed (sometimes cited as 40 weeks, sometimes 40 weeks plus 7 days, 40 weeks plus 10 days, or 42 weeks). In actual fact, going overdue is a matter of routine for most women, as the *Guide to Effective Care in Pregnancy and Childbirth* confirms: 'Post-term pregnancy, in most cases, probably represents a variant of normal, and is associated with a good outcome, regardless of the form of care given.'[5] Although many doctors cite increasing perinatal mortality rates at 42 weeks and beyond as a cast-iron reason for induction of labour, the truth is that clinical evidence does not support this notion unequivocally. Many women do go on to have normal births and healthy babies at 43 and even 44 weeks with the right preparation and support.

If your partner is overdue and her caregivers favour induction, then various methods may be suggested. The first may be a 'membrane sweep' or 'cervical sweep', whereby the midwife uses her fingers to gently open and 'sweep' around the cervix, separating the base of the baby's amniotic sac from the cervix and stimulating the release of natural labour hormones. This procedure has varying rates of success and may be relatively painless or extremely painful, depending on the practitioner's skill and your partner's emotional state. Regardless of these factors, a sweep can certainly be performed at home.

The next suggestion after the sweep is often pharmacological induction, whereby synthetic hormones are given (either as an intravenous drip or a vaginal pessary) to kick-start contractions. Often, it is suggested that a woman should have her waters broken as part of this process, so that the baby applies more direct pressure to the cervix. Either way, pharmacological induction must take place in a hospital, as careful monitoring is needed to make sure that mother and baby do not suffer an adverse reaction. This method of induction may cause contractions that are more erratic and painful than those that occur during spontaneous labour, and mothers and babies tolerate this intense uterine activity with varying levels of success.

In particular, a debate has begun to rage in clinical circles regarding the unlicensed use of misoprostol (commercially known as Cytotec) to induce labour. Originally intended as a treatment for ulcers, this drug gained popularity in the US when doctors realised that it could induce labour with unprecedented speed. However, research indicates that Cytotec can cause uterine hyperstimulation and even life-threatening uterine rupture in some women, particularly those who have had a previous Caesarean section. [6,7]

Moreover, with any kind of pharmacological induction, a woman's movement is often restricted while she receives IV drugs and wears the belt necessary to record data on the cardiotocograph (the monitor for fetal heartbeat and contractions). This restricted movement can have its own effects on the progress and comfort of labour, and may be one of the reasons why inductions are often associated with higher rates of forceps and Caesarean deliveries.[8]

Most midwives will support a home birth until 42 weeks of gestation, if not beyond. If your partner reaches 42 weeks, declines induction, and would still like to be attended at home after this point, she may wish to enquire about just how much practical and moral support she can expect for such a delivery. NHS midwives in some regions of the UK may not agree to a home birth after 42 weeks, although the women in their care are legally entitled to that assistance. Independent midwives in the UK and elsewhere may be more flexible; in any case, it is worth exploring this situation hypothetically well before it occurs in real life.

What can I do to help?

You and your partner may wish to decide how much faith to put in the EDD that you have been given and, in addition, whether you agree with your caregivers' definition of 'overdue'. It may be that you are both happy to wait until nature takes its course and labour begins spontaneously, no matter whether this happens at 40 or 43 weeks. If, however, the phone is ringing off the hook with eager well-wishers, the birth pool has begun gathering dust in the corner, and your partner is keen for labour to begin, then there are various natural methods of induction that you may wish to explore together. Many of these natural methods have their own staunch advocates and, as the days pass, no doubt you and your partner will be bombarded with 'fail-safe' techniques by friends, relatives and neighbours who are only too happy to share their own experiences. These techniques and tricks may include raspberry leaf tea, evening primrose oil, castor oil, fresh pineapple, spicy curries, long walks, sex, and nipple stimulation (yes, really). Complementary therapies, such as reflexology, acupuncture, and homeopathy, may offer more reliable results at this point. As with any intervention, your midwife may be able to provide you with more information, and you and your partner may wish to discuss the pros and cons of these methods before proceeding further.

If your partner has tried every natural remedy imaginable and is coming under increasing pressure to be induced by more clinical means, then you can discuss whether she might wish to be monitored more closely over the coming days. Investigations of placental function and of the amount of amniotic fluid around the baby may determine whether there is any realistic need to take action, providing reassurance to your partner and placating any overzealous doctors. This kind of monitoring may not be routinely offered, but it can be done on a day-patient basis at most hospitals.

The one thing you can certainly do with no ill effect is to reassure your partner of your faith in her and of your belief that your baby will arrive safely when the time is right. While these last few days may seem interminable, patience may be more of a virtue at this time than at any other.

What if labour goes on for days and days, and the baby just doesn't want to come out?

Your friends, neighbours and colleagues may already have regaled you with tales of their wives' Caesarean sections. 'Labour just seemed to be endless,' they say. 'We tried everything, and the baby just didn't want to come out,' they may sigh with expressions of sad resignation. Indeed, long labours with little apparent 'progress' in cervical dilation or fetal descent are the main reason for home-birthing women to transfer to a hospital and they are also the main indicator for Caesarean section across all births. Many parents feel disheartened by such an outcome, and when no real explanation is given by the medical caregivers in attendance, it may be easier to gloss over any existing questions or doubts with the blanket statement that 'the baby just didn't want to come out'.

This idea that a baby would not want to be born hardly holds up under scrutiny. Millions of years of evolution have conspired to make mother and baby perfectly suited for labour and birth in every way; the baby may be comfortable in the womb but its future survival does depend on its 'coming out' at some point.

While parents often blame the baby for a long and difficult birth, the medical establishment much prefers to blame the mother. When dilation and descent do not adhere to hospital protocols and timeframes, the words 'failure to progress' are writ large in a woman's notes. Never mind that she may have been subject to interventions such as a fetal heart monitor or an epidural that require her to lie on her back, thereby slowing down the natural course of her labour. Never mind that the hospital and the bedside manners of its employees may have caused the mother to tense up with anxiety or fear, interrupting the free flow of oxytocin. No, rather than examine their own procedures and practices, it is far easier for many medics to claim that the woman who now lies on the operating table has 'failed to progress'. If the mood takes them, they may elaborate on this diagnosis, attributing this woman's failure to her 'incoordinate uterus', 'incompetent cervix', or 'small pelvis'. In truth, the vast majority of women have pelvises, uteri, and cervices that are perfectly suited to the task at hand. Many mothers and midwives wonder whether 'failure to progress' would more aptly be called 'failure to wait'.

Even if babies really *do* want to come out and even if women aren't to blame, the question remains: why do some labours take so very long? As with virtually every aspect of birth, 'long' is a subjective concept. Hospitals may prefer women to dilate at a steady rate of one centimetre per hour, but your partner's cervix has no knowledge of the clock on the wall. Just as some women's labours are shockingly short sprints, those of some other women always seem to be marathons. As long as mother and baby are both well, 'long' can still be 'normal'.

What can I do to help?

In an ideal world, each baby would settle into its mother's pelvis in the optimal position, with head down, neck nicely flexed, and chin tucked snugly onto the chest. However, as any experienced parent knows, children don't always behave the way they should, and this rule applies from the very beginning of life. Babies nestle down for the journey of birth in all kinds of awkward positions: shoulders at a difficult angle, brow tilted up, body facing the wrong way; or rogue hands jammed up by the forehead, as if brushing away a stray lock of hair. In the majority of cases, these malpositions are adjusted by the movements of mother and baby during late pregnancy but, in some cases, they persist during labour and their resolution requires a bit of extra effort.

If labour seems to be taking a long time (and again, 'long' is subjective) with few apparent signs of progress, then it is possible that a slight malposition has slowed things down. You can encourage your partner to remain active, mobilising her pelvis in different ways and using gravity-effective positions. She can dance, lunge from one leg to the other, stand, squat, kneel, or walk up and down stairs. As you have prepared the birth space, you may be able to suggest different 'props' that your partner can use to experiment with different positions; she can lean over bean bags, chairs, the side of the bed or the kitchen counter. The buoyancy of water in the bath or birth pool can also help your partner to hold gravity-effective positions for longer. It should be noted that women who are unobserved will usually adopt the best positions for labour as a matter of instinct. If you sense that your partner feels a bit like her labour has become a spectator sport, then giving her some privacy for a while may well be the most helpful thing you can do.

If your partner appears to be exhausted after hours of effort, make sure that she is getting enough to eat and drink. Although hospitals often have a 'nil by mouth' rule during labour, dehydration and fatigue can actually cause more problems than such a policy might solve. Toast, cookies, energy bars, fruit (fresh or dried), squares of chocolate, spoonfuls of honey – all are easily digestible, energy-rich foods for labour. Water, fresh 'smoothies' and fruit juices are all good drinks at this time, although some midwives prefer isotonic sports drinks (such as Gatorade or Lucozade) since these drinks can restore vital calories and electrolytes without the potentially irritating acid of fruit juices. Your partner might not feel hungry or thirsty but, if she is fading fast, then even the tiniest nibble of toast or sip of juice may be enough to revive her. If she eats and drinks throughout labour, you might also like to remind her to visit the toilet every hour or so. A full bladder and/or bowel can impede the baby's descent, and the walk to and from the bathroom may also have the added benefit of settling the baby into a better position.

Sometimes no amount of dancing, jiggling, peeing or snacking can kick-start a sluggish labour. In these instances, it's possible that the mother's emotional state is the main hindrance to steady progress; tension, fear and desperation can prevent a woman from surrendering fully to her body's efforts. If your partner seems demoralised by the slow pace of events, then a change of location or atmosphere may be enough to lift her mood. You can suggest moving to a different room, listening to some upbeat music, opening the windows, or even going for a walk, if the weather permits. Laughter can be a powerful medicine; many labours have been known to accelerate after the telling of a particularly silly or saucy joke.

Sometimes a mother's troubles run so deep that neither knock-knock jokes nor funky music can touch them. Birth requires women to turn inwards for strength and, if that introspection reveals only turmoil and despair, then labour can grind to an almost irreversible halt. The process of 'letting go' – that total surrender which is so essential for a healthy birth – may be terrifying for any number of reasons. For some women, the powerful sensations of labour may arouse memories of abuse, assault, or previous traumatic births. Others may find themselves suddenly paralysed by lingering doubts about motherhood and the changes it will bring. There is no simple cure for this kind of emotional distress but you and your birth attendant(s) can gently ask your partner what she's thinking about, whether she's afraid of anything, and why. You can reassure her that she is safe, and that you will not allow anything or anyone to hurt her. She may not be able to conquer her fears on this occasion but, with the right support, she can acknowledge and move through them towards a joyful and healthy birth.

Whatever the reasons behind your partner's 'long' labour, it's worth remembering that you can only continue to provide your partner with valuable support if you are supported as well. A man who has not slept or eaten for days is of little use to his partner. You and the other members of your birth team can take turns staying with your partner while the weariest among you eats, sleeps, or simply gets a breath of fresh air. A half-hour catnap is better than none at all, and a peanut butter sandwich is better than crippling hunger. A little self-preservation will help you to greet your new baby – when he or she finally arrives – with a smile.

David N's Story
A long haul

David is an English chartered accountant whose hard-won faith in home birth was rewarded after his wife, Julia, soldiered through a long and difficult labour. His story shows how patience, confidence, and teamwork can be crucial during such arduous births.

Julia started her labour on the Friday afternoon/evening, by which time we were 11 days overdue and getting some pressure from our local midwife to go to hospital and see the specialist. At about 2am on Saturday morning, Julia woke me up and said that the contractions were becoming more frequent, so I was sent downstairs to light the wood-burner and make the house cosy. When I came back upstairs, I timed the contractions to be every 10 minutes. I started massaging Julia's back to help her with the pain, and at about 6am we contacted our doula, who arrived a few hours later.

We had both found it difficult to sleep, so that by the time our doula arrived, Julia and I were pleased that we had someone else to help provide support. It was such a relief to me when the doula arrived, as she helped to take the pressure off me, and as this was our doula's 26th birth, we knew we were in good hands. We had already agreed that a trainee doula could also come along, and she arrived around 10am.

From this point on, the doulas and I were able to share the provision of support to Julia, with constant massaging and encouragement. In addition, our doula was very good at sensing what would help Julia at different stages of the labour, such as moving to a small, dark room, or getting in the birth pool. At around 11am, our doula called the midwife, who arrived soon after and asked to examine Julia. This procedure was painful for Julia and it caused the labour to slow down, as we had thought might happen. But our doula was able to deal with this and she quickly got Julia back into the right mindset. The midwife identified that Julia was hardly dilated and that the baby was 'back-to-back' in spite of all of Julia's effort so far to try and turn the baby. We did not tell Julia this, as we did not want to demoralise her, and after the event, Julia was relieved that we hadn't told her about this at the time.*

* *Author's note:* When the baby's spine rests against the mother's spine in the 'back-to-back' or posterior position, labour can be longer and more challenging.

The midwife asked if she could leave and come back later, which we felt comfortable with, and the doulas and I got back to providing encouragement and support to Julia. Julia spent some more time in the birth pool, and I started running around and trying to keep everyone going: making meals, drinks, etc., and answering the phone when Julia's mother called. I told her that Julia had gone out and would phone her back later! By mid-afternoon, it was getting hard for me to keep going and I am sure that I was starting to get demoralised from seeing Julia in so much pain, for so long, and with so little obvious progress. I was tired, and trying to be so supportive to Julia for so long was mentally exhausting (although nothing compared to what Julia was going through).

Our midwife returned around 3pm and asked to examine Julia again. Julia reluctantly agreed, and the midwife announced that Julia was now about six centimetres dilated. Unfortunately, our midwife was now coming towards the end of her shift, but she assured us that she would get another excellent midwife to do the actual delivery. Fortunately, our doula knew most of the local midwives and she assured us that the replacement midwife was also very good.

The new midwife arrived at around 4pm, and at first I was a bit concerned, as she was a lot younger and quieter than the first midwife, and she didn't immediately put me at ease. However, as the birth progressed, we discovered that these concerns were totally unfounded.

By around 4pm, the pain was starting to get unbearable for Julia, and the midwife offered gas and air. This immediately brought fantastic relief for Julia and enabled her to continue through to the delivery. I am not sure that Julia would have been able to continue at this point if it hadn't been for this intervention. By that time, Julia was back in the birth pool; she felt most comfortable there and she had decided to have the baby in the water, if possible.

One of Julia's greatest fears was the risk of tearing during the actual delivery and she was keen to avoid this if at all possible. After hours and hours of pushing, the midwife told Julia not to stop pushing with the contractions, but to relax during each one in order to allow the baby effectively to push itself out. This was so difficult, but the midwife was superb at helping Julia; we were all very impressed by just how good the midwife was at handling this situation.

Once the baby's head was through, Julia was able to feel it in the water. I had decided that I didn't want to see the baby coming out, so I positioned myself behind Julia to provide massage and support. I just wanted to have my first memory of our baby as being complete, rather than just part of him showing.

At 5.38pm, the baby was born. Julia lifted him out of the water and held him up to her chest so that his head was just above her left shoulder and his face was only a few inches from mine. I saw him open his eyes and look into mine, and then he looked around for a few seconds as if to say, 'Where am I? This doesn't look like it did the last time I opened my eyes!' I will never forget that moment when we first saw each other, and I first looked at my son. After a few minutes, he had still not started breathing, so the midwife advised that she should cut the cord and do whatever was needed to start his breathing. We agreed to this, even though we had said in our birth plan that we wanted to let the cord pulse for longer. At 5.41pm, Jonathan started breathing after a rub with a towel.

Julia got out of the pool at this point, as she wanted to deliver the placenta naturally. I took off my shirt and held Jonathan close to my chest so that he could hear my heartbeat and feel my warmth. He cried a little at first, but he soon stopped when he heard the familiar sound of my heartbeat. I'm sure that he recognised my voice, as I had spoken to him often when he was still in the womb.

David H's Story

Giggles, roars, and a baby

David is a production engineer from England whose two children were both born at home. The following story describes his first baby's arrival, and illustrates the importance of keeping faith in the natural process of labour even if things appear to have slowed or stalled.

The 40 weeks leading up to Oliver's birth were all pretty stress-free and easy for us to cope with. Helen didn't have any sickness, no massive bump, and no swollen ankles. She was just a crotchety woman who wanted a few pints!

The due date was set for February 14. That date came and went, although I wasn't at all surprised. The baby was having a great time in there! On February 17 at about 10pm, we decided it was time to go to bed. The usual routine, brushing teeth and a short conversation, agreeing that we would make the most of our Saturday morning lie-in tomorrow, in case it was our last one. We certainly got that right. Within minutes of saying this, Helen's waters started to leak. Not a gush like we had imagined, but a small trickle.

So, we went to bed (Helen with a towel underneath). Every time Helen got up to go to the toilet, more water would come out . . . and then the contractions started. I was given a blow-by-blow account of each contraction and each leak. Helen was really excited, and a giggling buffoon. I suggested that she get back into bed and to go to sleep for a bit.

I was just slipping off to sleep when I was nudged to be told that the contractions were regular, lasting about one minute, and could I put the TENS machine on? Helen also insisted that we should call the midwife. Because the contractions were only three minutes apart, birth wasn't a million miles away (or so Helen thought).

The midwife came out at midnight and she was really supportive. Every contraction that Helen had was followed by a giggle, so I think I realised that this was not established labour, and a baby was not about to appear before our eyes! So I went back to sleep whilst Helen took refuge on the toilet, and the midwife went away again.

Come the morning, we called the midwife out at about 9.30am. She came along, and by this stage, Helen had moved downstairs to the middle room – this was going to be the 'action room', where we wanted our baby to be born. We'd even put up blacked-out polythene at the windows and moved the dining room table out to mark the occasion. After an examination, the midwife informed Helen that she was about four centimetres dilated. We wondered if we might have our baby by lunchtime, then.

Helen laboured on, and all of the things that she had thought she would want during her labour – such as lots of massaging, stroking, talking, etc. – were the last things she wanted. This made me quite redundant, really. All I could do was to be there and obey instructions if given.

It was around about mid-morning that Helen needed a bit more analgesic help. So she started on the old entonox. This was where I came to the fore. With every contraction, it was my job to hold the mouthpiece to her mouth.

Helen would take a big breath of it in. And so it went on . . . I remember glancing at the clock periodically – hours just seemed to tick by with nothing else much happening.

Helen had another examination. It was established that she was still at four centimetres. I could see that she was absolutely gutted at this point, feeling rather tired, and just wanting the birth bit to happen. When Helen was asked when she had last 'had a wee', we realised that it must have been hours ago. So another one of my important roles was to accompany Helen to the toilet and encourage her to wee! She was told that she would probably have to turn the TENS machine off for this, which she did, but she very quickly turned it back on again! She was terrified about turning it off, as it seemed to be helping her so much. I put a lot of effort into encouraging urination, but unfortunately, none happened. In the end, it took a catheter, and a litre and a half of urine later, Helen's labour started to progress again.

Everything seemed quite calm; we just dealt with each contraction as it presented itself. It was probably around this time, after a bit of a desperate moment, that Helen asked, 'Please help me!' Afterwards, Helen told me that she had been struggling with some negative thoughts, and was really worried that they would want to transfer us to hospital.

Then Helen decided that she really wanted to be in the bathroom, so we had to up sticks and transfer everything upstairs. This is where we remained from about 4pm onwards. It was at this point that Helen started to make noises I'd never heard a human make before. Guttural and animal-like. This was second stage labour! At last, I thought, this was the end. Any minute now, a baby would appear.

But oh no – there were two more hours of this. I could see Helen getting weaker and weaker, and at some points, her contractions started to dry up. They were dropping to every five minutes and the intensity had dropped considerably. Helen was on all fours, leaning over the birthing ball and facing me. I could see the midwives looking at each other after each contraction and shaking their heads, as if to say 'no good'. I continued to give Helen lots of positive comments but I couldn't help but feel apprehensive.

Then finally, the baby's head started to crown. I could now see the top of our baby's head. At 6.04pm, Oliver eventually slid out. Hallelujah! Weighing in at 8 lbs and perfect in every way, just a very bruised-looking nose and a Vulcan-shaped head - a testimony to the long labour.[*]

We decided not to cut the cord for some time, about 20 minutes in all. After the placenta had been delivered and the midwives had cleared up and left us, we just couldn't stop staring at Oliver. We stared more, and then some more. And we haven't really stopped staring since.

What if the baby arrives before the midwife does?

Here, a mother-to-be begins to answer that question:

> *Then all of a sudden I said 'I'm pushing,' then I felt stupid – how could I be when I wasn't in labour? Even if I was in labour, it was too early to be pushing, it had only started an hour ago. Tony started panicking. I said, 'It's okay, I'm not pushing, I'm pooing.' He said 'That's a very hairy poo!'*[9]

Most of the time, Mother Nature gives a woman a fair bit of advance warning that her baby is on the way. However, on the rare occasion when

---

[*] *Author's note:* it is not unusual for babies to emerge with slightly misshapen heads if they have been pushing against the cervix in an awkward or asymetrical position over a long period of time. Such moulding is not dangerous, as the plates of babies' skulls are somewhat loose and pliable to aid their passage through the pelvis, and the apparent deformity usually disappears within hours or days.

active labour is exceptionally brief, even the best prepared mother is caught on the hop. 'Twinges' quickly turn into contractions, which morph with lightning speed into pushes, and hey presto, there's a baby (or a 'hairy poo', as in the story above). These wham-bam-thank-you-ma'am experiences are known as 'precipitous births', with active labour over in three hours or less. The term couldn't be more apt: for many parents, the sudden realisation that a baby is about to arrive is accompanied by the same dizzying rush that comes with leaping from a 'precipice' high above the ground. Before you've had the chance to think about jumping, you've already been pushed.

While the prospect of a precipitous birth with no midwife in sight might be terrifying for some parents, the speed of the event does not necessarily indicate a commensurate level of danger. 'Such births usually have good outcomes, wherever they take place,' notes midwife Ina May Gaskin. 'Mother and baby survive, often to the amazement of the general public, which has been systematically – if not deliberately – brainwashed over the last century or so to fear childbirth.'[10] Indeed, a large proportion of the non-hospital birth stories that appear in the media seem to follow the theme that Gaskin describes: mother has a slight case of 'indigestion', mother suddenly finds herself pushing, mother reaches down to feel a baby's head hanging out of her body, and mother births her baby on the bathroom floor / in a taxi on the way to the hospital / by the side of the road. The baby's safe arrival is always greeted with shock and effusive gratitude, and many such stories conclude with the mother's insistence that she 'couldn't have done it without' the neighbour / taxi driver / passer-by who assisted her. The truth is much simpler than these stories would have us believe: precipitous births have been happening for as long as women have been having babies and for the most part, they are just another variation of 'normal'. Kindly neighbours and taxi drivers may be helpful, but women are the world's experts on birthing their own babies.

What can I do to help?

Different men have different responses to the immortal words, 'The baby's coming – NOW!' That statement strikes fear deep into the hearts of many men, who may always have imagined themselves playing a somewhat more peripheral role in labour and birth. For others, the realisation that they are about to experience birth in its most intimate, immediate form is an adrenaline rush like no other – 'the go-for-it feeling', as one father puts it. As a home-birthing father, you do not have to worry about making the trip to hospital as your wife valiantly tries to cross her legs in the back of the car. You can rest easy in the knowledge that you are already in the place that you have chosen for the safe birth of your baby, even if that birth is happening with a speed that you could never have predicted.

One of the first things you might want to think about when birth seems imminent is what kind of medical assistance you may be able to find at the last minute. If you have an independent midwife, then do you have time to call her, and can she talk you through the birth over the phone? If you are working with a hospital-based midwifery team, then do you want to phone the hospital's labour suite? If you answer yes to the latter, then there is a chance that a midwife at the hospital will be able to talk you through events as they unfold, but there is also a chance that she will advise you to call an ambulance, or that she will insist on sending one herself. The arrival of paramedics instantly transforms your baby's birth into an 'emergency situation', a diagnosis with which you and your partner may or may not concur. Even if, and perhaps especially if, your partner is in the final throes of labour, it is important that you and she agree whether or not such measures are warranted.

If medical help is nowhere to be seen and it's clear that you'll be playing the role of baby catcher, then the best thing you can do is to stay calm. Easier said than done, of course, but as with any birth, your attitude can have a major effect on your partner's comfort and self-confidence. You may not have expected this situation, but it's happening, and no amount of panic can change that. Remind your partner (and yourself) that she is doing wonderfully, that she is strong, that you love her, and that birth is a safe, normal process.

Any suggestions to 'hold it in' or 'just hang on until the midwife gets here' may be met with a distinctly frosty response; indeed, if your partner truly feels that the baby is about to be born, then all three of you are now passengers on an unstoppable train. The only thing to do is to go along for the ride and, if possible, enjoy the view. Encourage your partner to follow her urges to bear down when she wants to bear down, and to breathe when she needs to breathe. If your partner is overwhelmed by the strength of her contractions, then she may want to try lying on her side or going onto all fours, with her head resting on her hands. However, bear in mind that most women spontaneously assume the position that is most comfortable and effective for them.

In terms of practical preparations, you should ensure that the room is warm and that there are clean towels and blankets nearby. Your partner may wish to catch the baby herself, or she may prefer you to do so; either way, it might be wise to prepare a soft 'landing pad' of pillows or towels under your partner in case the baby emerges at top speed. If you are taking instructions from a midwife over the phone, try to describe clearly what you can see so that the midwife can offer advice accordingly.

Supporting skin-to-skin contact immediately after birth has been shown to provide babies with a number of short- and long-term benefits, from improved regulation of heartbeat and body temperature to decreased crying and longer duration of breastfeeding.[11] You might like to wrap the baby (and your partner) in a clean towel or blanket as they have their first cuddle. If the first feed hastens the delivery of the placenta, then you can simply leave the umbilical cord intact and place the placenta in a bowl or wrap it in a towel until medical assistance arrives. Do not attempt to cut the cord yourself.

If mother and baby are well, you can pause to enjoy a sense of intimacy and accomplishment that few parents get to experience. A precipitous birth can be a shock, but it can also be an event of incomparable joy, as this baby-catching father explains:

> *Seeing my wife give birth to my daughter in such an intimate environment was absolutely the most exciting and emotionally exhilarating experience that I have ever had. I just can't describe the depth of love that I felt and the feeling of pride that soon followed. This was a huge accomplishment for us. I caught my children as they entered the world. Nothing can bring a father closer to his child than that. (Kevin)*

David H's Story
'Tell me how to stop it!'

The arrival of David and Helen's second child was an altogether quicker affair than the birth of their first child, Oliver, less than a year before. Although Helen had some gentle early twinges over the course of several days, a few powerful contractions soon tipped the balance.

Daisy's due date was 28 February, 2006. Helen, my wife, had a perfect pregnancy and felt fit and well throughout. Tiredness was a bit of an issue because she was looking after Oliver, who was under the age of one at the time, but we are a good team, which made it all the easier.

On Friday, 23 February, Helen had a show. This is not something she had experienced with Oliver. After checking with other girlfriends that it actually was a show, we started really looking forward to what would soon be coming our way again.

Helen had the usual Friday with Oliver. They went to the toddler group at the Methodist Church. Helen was having mild contractions every 35-45 minutes but she told me that all of these pre-labour signs could last for at least a week.

The next day, we had a normal Saturday. Walked into Worcester for coffee and cakes. The contractions still continued and we were wondering whether anything was going to happen. Later that day, Helen decided she was going to see the local homeopath for some Caulophyllum. He explained that it helped tone the uterine muscles and ripen the cervix. For the rest of the afternoon, we watched the England v. Scotland match whilst Helen bounced away on her birth ball.

That night, we planned to have steak for dinner. But as the contractions were regularly occurring every 20 minutes or so, we decided that pasta would be a much better idea, just in case more was destined to happen that evening.

We bathed Oliver, and just as I was about to put him to bed, Helen decided that he should really go to Granny and Grandad's. Things, she thought, were definitely going to happen. So the poor little chap was hurried off to Granny and Grandad's in his pyjamas.

After our pasta dinner, I spent the evening watching some ridiculous television (at Helen's request). She just bounced away on her birth ball and asked me to hook her up to the TENS machine. We had practised this a few times, so I knew where the pads should more or less go.

Helen's contractions were still quite far apart, but definitely getting stronger. She said that the rubbish she was forcing me to watch on the television was a good distraction. In between bouncing on the birth ball, Helen made sure that she kept active, making many trips up and down to the toilet! At around 10pm, I decided that I was going to go to bed. It wasn't an easy decision to make, but I thought that we would have hours and hours ahead of us, and it was important for me to get some rest too. Helen was not at all happy with this decision. She used every stalling technique known to keep me with her, even sitting on top of me to prevent me from going upstairs! I realised that she was dead serious. So maybe something was going to happen ...

After Helen's umpteenth trip to the toilet, she reappeared looking a bit concerned. I decided that it was time to call the midwife. I put the call into Ambulance Control (to page the midwife) whilst Helen disappeared upstairs again. She reappeared back downstairs fairly swiftly and asked me if the midwife was coming. We realised that this baby was going to arrive – very soon! I made another call to Ambulance Control to check that the midwife was on her way over, and they said that she was.

Helen had relocated to the dining room at this point with her birth ball. She told me that she would try the 'brace position' she had been taught in yoga. But to no avail. Before I knew it, I heard the guttural noise of second-stage labour, which I remembered from our birth with Oliver.

I asked Helen if she wanted me to 'have a look'. She said no but I did anyway, and for sure, I could see the top of this baby's head. I got back onto Ambulance Control and told them what was happening. They told me that they would have to talk me through it all on the phone. I just wanted them to tell me how to stop it, but there was no going back.

With the next contraction, the baby was crowning. I supported the baby's head to help ease the pressure. I then had to put the phone down on the floor to go for the catch! I saw the baby's head come out and then it turned so that the shoulders followed, just as we had learnt in our antenatal classes. Thankfully, I caught her perfectly. A baby girl.

The ambulance controller was absolutely brilliant. 'Is the baby breathing?,' she asked. I repeated the question to Helen because I was unsure of the answer, but as Daisy was starting to scream, we realised that yes, she was indeed breathing. I passed her up to Helen and we wrapped her in a towel and started to dry her off. She just looked so tiny.

We then heard the clip-clop of the midwife's shoes coming down the passageway. We were so happy to see her! 'Oh, you didn't need me,' she said as she came in. We were just about to discuss the third stage of birth when nature answered the question for us – plop! Out came the placenta and sploshed onto the floor. Mmmm, lovely. So I spent the next two hours trying to get the blood stain out of the floor – we were in the process of selling our house and had a viewing arranged for the next day!

All in all, it was probably the most incredible experience of my life. There surely isn't a better place to be born than into your Daddy's hands.

Kevin's Story
Awe and disbelief

As a computer network operations manager in Texas, Kevin had little opportunity to practise his baby-catching skills prior to his daughter's arrival. However, in spite of this relative inexperience, Kevin kept a cool head when the birth picked up pace – even when it became clear that the baby had her cord around her neck, and her hand by her face.

It was eight o'clock in the evening when Crystal started having contractions. Not Braxton Hicks, but real contractions. Knowing that our midwife, Bonnie, was more than fifty minutes away, I asked Crystal if we should call her, but Crystal insisted that the contractions were too mild, and that she wanted to let Bonnie get some rest. She assumed that this would be a long, drawn-out labour and that Bonnie would have plenty of time.

A few hours passed and the contractions continued with a similar consistency. By 11 o'clock, they were about five minutes apart, lasting 35 to 45 seconds, but still bearably mild. Crystal had taken a bath as she insisted on shaving her legs, stopping for contractions and then continuing on with the strokes until she was smooth and 'presentable'. I asked several times if I should call the midwife, and Crystal still insisted that the contractions were too mild. Finishing her bath and preparing to blow-dry her hair, she finally decided to take a break and go to bed.

While Crystal had been in the bath, our friend Stephanie and I had prepared the bed with a plastic mattress liner, two sets of sheets, and other 'no mess' items. When she got out of the tub, I had sterilised it with bleach. We'd already put a few blankets on the bathroom floor, too. Crystal hadn't wanted to commit to a single location for the birth, so we now had three different options in place.

At 11.45pm, Crystal finally suggested that I call Bonnie and ask her to come out, which I did. By midnight, Crystal asked that I call Bonnie again and tell her to hurry. Bonnie was on her way, but her cell phone was out of signal, and it went straight to voice mail. Crystal got out of bed and went to sit on the toilet. I was on my knees in front of her to comfort her during contractions. Well, she had two contractions on the toilet that were less than two minutes apart, and strong.

During the second contraction, we heard a splash into the toilet – Crystal's waters had broken and the fluid rushed into the toilet. We both looked at each other like, 'What was that?'; but at the same time we knew what had happened. The next contraction came very quickly when Crystal said, 'I have to push.'

I looked around, and I was the only one there. Stephanie was in the spare room, but I didn't have a second to leave and get her to help. I remember thinking, 'Oh my God, I'm going to deliver this baby by myself,' and immediately after, I thought, 'Cool, we are going to have this baby intimately, by ourselves.' This was a thought that I began to cherish. Just then, Crystal said, 'I feel the head,' and I could hear the pain in her voice. I reached my hand between her legs. I don't know what I was thinking except that I might be able to catch it if it were to fall into the toilet. She quickly yelled at me to get my hand out of there.

'Crystal, you're not having this baby on the toilet,' I said as she finished off that contraction. Apparently she agreed, as she quickly leaned forward off the toilet and onto her hands and knees, hugging the edge of the tub. With three blankets down and towels nearby, I was thankful that we had prepared the floor. At that time, I was able to get a good view of what was going on down there. Crystal was yelling at the top of her lungs and I could see the head beginning to crown. There was this plentifully dark-haired scalp working its way out. Again, I looked around – still, just me.

The pain must have been intense, because Crystal was yelling so loud that I was expecting the police to come knocking on my door. (They're just down the street, you know!) When her contraction finished, the head was partially out and I could see parts of baby Aubrey's forehead. I asked Crystal to try and relax and prepare to push during the next contraction. I was surprised that she actually agreed and didn't yell at me.

I have never felt anything so intense. I was scared to death, worried that I might not be able to go through with this, and at the same time, excited and in control. The thought had crossed my mind a number of times about complications and how to deal with them. I didn't have time analyse every possibility; I prayed for a smooth delivery and continued on.

The next contraction came within a minute, and with a push, I was able to see the baby's eyes. I told Crystal that she was facing up and in the right position, and that most of her head was out. I knew that the next contraction would deliver the whole head. There was barely enough room, but I gently worked my finger into the vagina to search for the cord. I figured that if there were to be a complication at this time, the cord would be it. Sure enough, I found the cord around the baby's neck. I told Crystal and asked her what I should do. I was surprised when she very calmly told me to take the cord and pull it over the baby's head. I tried that, but it was too tight, so I held it off of her neck until the next contraction. Crystal gave a big push and Aubrey's head came out in full view. At that time, I was able to reposition the cord.

While feeling for the cord, I had also noticed that Aubrey's left hand was up by her face. Her hand didn't come out with her head. Crystal had asked if a shoulder was out, and I told her no. I assured her that it would be next. I gently reached my finger in again and felt her shoulder. With the next contraction, I was able to assist the left shoulder and hand out. The right shoulder followed almost immediately.

Within seconds, and without any further resistance, a perfect beautiful baby had fallen out of my wife and into my hands. I could hear Crystal's sigh of relief, and then she told me to get a towel and wipe our new baby off. When I began to towel her, our baby took her first breath. She was seconds old, still blue and in my hands. At 12.20am, she entered our lives.

Crystal turned around and I handed our new baby to her. We both wept and sat in awe and disbelief. I felt a huge sense of relief; Crystal and I had successfully brought our daughter into the world.

Reality set in as I started to relive what had just happened. I began to hyperventilate and started getting dizzy, but I quickly got over it. Crystal and I were both so overwhelmed that we failed to even check the sex until Stephanie came into the bathroom to see the new arrival.

What about that cord? Crystal insisted that we had to wait for the midwife before we dealt with it. Shortly after the birth, I called Bonnie again to tell her what had happened – she was on her way, and asked a few questions to check up on Crystal and Aubrey.

Stephanie and I helped Crystal to bed; we took pictures, and wrapped the baby in a nice warm blanket and a beanie cap. After about ten minutes, Crystal said it was time to birth the placenta. We grabbed a bowl and placed it on the bed as Crystal climbed out of bed and squatted. The placenta quickly dropped into the bowl. Again, and I asked about cutting the cord, and again, Crystal assured me that it was OK to wait for Bonnie.

So there we were: our birth was perfect, our baby was perfect, Crystal was doing great, and we had successfully delivered our child without any assistance. To this day, I feel a great sense of pride in knowing that our baby girl was delivered into my hands – a feat that any man would be proud to call his own.

Alan's Story

'I'd have gone through a wall'

Several years after Alan and Leah's first daughter was born by Caesarean section, the couple conceived again and decided to plan for a more peaceful, natural birth at home. Their HBAC (home birth after Caesarean) plans were greeted with reactions ranging from scepticism to shock but, as the following story illustrates, the birth couldn't have been more straightforward.

During our first daughter's birth in hospital, I felt that Leah and I had no control over the situation. After a couple of hours in, I didn't even have any confidence in the midwife – she was just treating my wife's labour like a factory job, like Leah was a battery hen. As things progressed, surgeons and various people came in and examined her, offering no explanation whatsoever, and then Leah was carted away for an emergency section. I was sent to change into my gown in a cleaners' cupboard with another guy who was waiting for his wife; the two of us couldn't speak to each other because we were both shell-shocked. After that horrible experience, I wanted to be able to give Leah the opportunity to have the birth she deserved. In a way, I was lucky to have been involved in such a piss-poor, unprofessional act on my wife, because then the idea of having a home birth didn't faze me; having the baby in a park would have been better than what we went through.

Finally, we conceived again. A week before Leah was due, I was at my parents' house about half an hour from home; our daughter, Sasha, was with me too. Leah phoned me in the afternoon and told me that her waters had broken, so I rushed home with Sasha in the car. I felt sheer excitement – the adrenaline was pumping up, and I'd have gone through a wall at that point. I had a real capable feeling, like I was about to go and serve, like a troop being called up, or somebody going over the top of a trench.

When I got home, Leah's waters had gone a bit more but she still hadn't felt any contractions. I started vacuuming and washing dishes so the place would be tidy for the midwives coming. I think Leah wanted to be on her own, so she went upstairs to the bedroom with the stereo, some oils, and a newspaper – we thought it would still be a long time before anything really happened. Leah came downstairs once or twice, but the main thing was focusing on what she needed or wanted to do, to try as much as I could not to bombard her with any questions. I just let her give me instructions.

I think I realised Leah was in labour when I went upstairs and she was already on her hands and knees on the bed, doing real deep groaning, a deep baritone moan or a wail – it was a sound different from anything I'd heard during Sasha's birth. She seemed well in control of it. I went and phoned the doula to ask her to come, and I took Sasha to our neighbours next door. By the time I came back upstairs, Leah was getting more into things, and I knew she was in a place that she hadn't been to before; I knew this time was different.

Leah started touching down below because she thought that maybe she could feel something there, and time started accelerating quickly at that point; maybe it had been an hour and a half since I'd gotten home. The doula hadn't turned up yet, so I phoned her back to see what was happening there, and then I phoned the midwives at the hospital. The midwife that was meant to come couldn't be contacted or paged for some reason, so they were sending out another two midwives.

I was on the phone to another midwife in the labour suite from that point, right up until the birth. She was asking me questions like what Leah was doing, what she sounded like, could I see anything, etc. Leah was still on her hands and knees and I could start to see the ridge of the baby's head. Leah had basically shut herself off from the world and was doing what she needed to do to get herself and the baby through the situation. My world just became passing information about what I was seeing to this woman on the phone, who was really good and really calm.

As things kept progressing, the midwife on the phone said she'd have to send an ambulance crew to the house. I told Leah and Leah said no, but the midwife said, 'No, it's protocol, we have to send them.' More of the head was showing at that point and the midwife was telling me to be prepared to check for a cord around the neck and to get the baby up straight away and onto Leah's body as quick as I could.

Then the ambulance crew turned up, and that was weird. When I saw them from the window, they were mucking about outside their motor and there was no rush to come in. That was fine, I wasn't panicking, but seeing them turn up was just a distraction. I had to leave Leah to open the door at a moment when I didn't want to leave her; then the paramedics came in and I didn't even want to talk to them because I knew that Leah didn't want to talk to them. They came upstairs and one of them stood in the hall – he didn't even want to come in. I got back on the phone and the midwife asked me, 'Do you want to hand over to the paramedics, or do you want to stay where you are?', and I said I wanted to stay where I was.

The paramedic that did come in was asking daft questions like how far apart the contractions were and when Leah's waters had broken, but the baby's head was sitting right there and it was obviously an alien situation to this guy; he was out of his depth. Straight away, I could see the panic in his face, and the other guy still didn't want to come into the room.

To my eyes, I could see that Leah was just one big push away from giving birth to our baby. What I could see was an absolutely amazing thing, an animalistic sort of strength, like a sprinter about to go out of the blocks – Leah showed total physical ability and control. She could easily have just been alone in that room and she'd have delivered a perfect baby and done everything herself. The midwife on the phone had said we'd need assistance, but I knew Leah didn't need any help.

I caught the baby: she came out to the head and shoulders, and then kind of slackened, and then the rest of her just kind of slid out into my hands. As the baby slid out the last bit, she came right round to me, and I remember turning her a wee bit and the cord kind of slipped off her shoulder, so there was no problem. I wrapped her in a clean towel I'd prepared, and then when a load of blood and stuff came out as well, in my nature, I put a clean towel on the bed to cover up the mess!

The midwives had come in just as I caught the baby, and they started to get more involved. They tried to settle Leah round, although she wasn't ready to hold the baby just yet. I could see she was busy with a bit of self-preservation; I knew straight away that she was fine, but that she'd been through a physically challenging thing and just needed a few moments to back off and check herself out. The midwives suggested that I get the baby onto my chest, so I pulled my T-shirt off. As they put the baby onto me, I remember her instantly trying to go for my nipple!

The midwives began chatting to the ambulance men, not chatting to me or Leah in our own house, which I thought was a bit strange. They said we needed to get Leah's placenta out, so it was more pushing for Leah, which I could clearly see she didn't want to do yet. I remember them saying to the paramedics, 'Do you want to see this placenta come out, and then you can say you've done the whole birth?', and I thought, 'That's crazy, he's going to go home and put in his log book that he's delivered a baby tonight.' I wasn't even going to say I'd delivered a baby, because my wife delivered a baby that night! In any case, the placenta came eventually, the baby snuggled in for a good feed, and everything was fine. The doula arrived, and she blended right in; it was great to have somebody there just to look after Leah.

To go from everybody trying to do everything for us in the hospital to us being able to do everything ourselves at home was absolutely amazing. It was, without a doubt, the peak experience of my life.

What if the baby becomes distressed?

During the first stage of labour, the midwife will monitor your baby's heartbeat at least every fifteen minutes once she has begun her partogram (heart rate chart). During the second stage (pushing), she will listen in with increasing frequency. A healthy baby usually has a heart rate between 120 and 160 beats per minute, although babies' 'baseline' rates can vary somewhat within that range. One of the most important things the midwife will be assessing is whether the baby's heart copes well with contractions: a healthy baby will show some variability within the normal range, reacting to and recovering from its mother's exertions as labour progresses.

There are a few heart patterns that may cause the midwife some concern. Heart rates that rise and fall dramatically, those that appear fairly 'flat' with little variability, those which remain consistently high, and those which dip at a contraction's peak and return sluggishly to normal at its end may require more careful monitoring over time.

What can I do to help?

There is little you can do to influence your baby's heart rate. However, in the first instance after a worrisome heart tone, you or the midwife might suggest to your partner that she change position. Occasionally, a baby's umbilical cord can become pinched or compressed in the pelvis, and a bit of movement can solve the problem by freeing the cord. If the midwife fails to be reassured by subsequent checks over a period of time, then the baby may not be coping well with labour and transfer to hospital may be appropriate.

What if the baby is born with the cord around its neck?

Many home birth sceptics ask this question, perhaps imagining that such a scenario might require a 'code red' hospital emergency with frantic doctors and the use of highly specialised machinery. In reality, it is not uncommon for a baby to be born with its umbilical cord around its neck, and the solution to this problem is fairly commonplace as well: in most cases, the cord is loose enough to allow the midwife to slip it back over the baby's head so that the rest of the body can be born.

In rare instances where the cord is too short or too tightly wound to be lifted, the midwife may need to cut and clamp the cord before the rest of the baby emerges. Because the baby will no longer be receiving oxygen from its cord, the midwife will want to ensure that the baby is delivered and helped to breathe on its own soon afterwards. There are a number of ways to encourage a baby to take its first breaths, such as blowing across her face, tickling the soles of her feet, or massaging her gently. If these measures are unsuccessful, then other techniques might be used to stimulate breathing: mucus can be suctioned from the baby's nose and mouth, more vigorous massage can be applied, and an 'ambu-bag' (oxygen bag) can be used. Every midwife who attends a home birth should have the training and equipment necessary for these basic resuscitation techniques.

What can I do to help?

The best you can do in this situation is to stay calm, trust in your baby's strength, and have faith in the skill of your midwife. If the midwife has to take a few moments to assist your baby's breathing, you can still stay close to your partner and offer her your support and reassurance until the baby can be handed safely to her for skin-to-skin contact.

What if my partner tears during birth?

Many gentle, physiological births result in little or no tearing of the perineum (the stretchy tissue between the vagina and the anus). Those tears that do occur are often minor and may heal well on their own without stitching. Your midwife should feel competent in administering local anaesthetic and suturing first- or second-degree tears, if need be. In the rare instance of a third-degree tear (involving deep muscle tissues as well as perineal skin), a trip to the hospital may be in order.

What can I do to help?

Prevention is often the best cure for perineal tears. Some midwives recommend a late-pregnancy programme of perineal massage, which has been shown to offer a slight reduction of trauma to this delicate area during birth, particularly in mothers who have not given birth vaginally before.[12] Such massage involves inserting a finger or two and gently stretching the tissues around the base and sides of the vagina, often with the aid of a neutral oil such as wheatgerm or olive oil. Your partner may invite you to join her in this routine. However, your eagerness to 'lend a hand' may be met with shock, hilarity, or worse. Rest assured that perineal massage is not for everyone, and it is certainly not a prerequisite for a safe birth.

During the first stage of labour, your partner might like to minimise her risk of tearing by labouring in water, which helps tissues to soften naturally over time. When the second stage begins and it's time to push, some midwives use warm compresses to aid the softening process, while others simply keep a watchful eye on the perineum, perhaps suggesting a few well-timed 'pants' rather than pushes if the tissues appear to be stretched dangerously thin. There is little that you can do at this point apart from encouraging your partner to follow her natural instincts; she knows best how to birth this baby in her own time.

What if my partner loses too much blood during or after the birth?

When some people think of home birth, they imagine a scene of blood-spattered horror that would be more appropriate to *The Texas Chainsaw Massacre* than the gentle arrival of a baby. In actual fact, most women lose about 500 millilitres of blood or less around the time of birth – just about enough to fill a small saucepan. Any bleeding beyond that amount may qualify as a haemorrhage and may require medical intervention in your home or, in more extreme cases, in the hospital.

One of the main causes of excessive blood loss during labour is placenta praevia, a condition in which the placenta lies low enough to touch or even cover the cervix. As labour progresses and the baby's head moves down, the placenta may become partially or fully separated from the uterus, causing blood loss and immediate danger to both mother and baby. You may be reassured to know that placenta praevia affects only a very small percentage of births because the condition is fairly rare and most low-lying placentas are detected during antenatal ultrasound scans. If a woman is found, during pregnancy, to have a dangerously low placenta, then her healthcare providers may well recommend a Caesarean section; or, at the very least, a trial of labour in the hospital.

Postpartum haemorrhage (PPH) is excessive bleeding that occurs after the birth itself. It is more common than placenta praevia, but it is still only thought to affect a relatively small proportion of all births. A certain amount of blood loss is to be expected when the placenta separates from the uterine wall, but the blood vessels usually contract in response to the body's own oxytocin (or, in the 'active management' style of delivery, a synthetic oxytocic drug). If, for whatever reason, the blood vessels do not contract, then continuous blood loss can occur and swift action must be taken.

It's impossible to make any early and reliable predictions about which women will experience PPH, although a midwife will be able to identify certain risk factors that might predispose your partner to such a bleed, such as a clotting disorder, pre-eclampsia (a syndrome involving pregnancy-induced high blood pressure), pregnancy with twins, or, for women who have already had at least one baby, a short interval between this pregnancy and the last. As a home-birthing father, you can take comfort in the fact that some of the greatest risk factors of PPH are hospital-based procedures such as induction of labour, Caesarean section, and other surgical interventions.

What can I do to help?

The midwife will monitor your partner carefully for any signs of excessive blood loss, and if haemorrhage is suspected, she will be able to take immediate action. Deep tears will be identified and stitched, if possible; an oxytocic drug will be given to encourage the contraction of the uterine blood vessels, if this has not already been administered; the midwife might also massage your partner's uterus to assist the contraction process; and she might call an ambulance with a request for further assistance en route to the hospital. An intravenous drip of fluids may be required and, in rare cases of true PPH, a blood transfusion may be necessary.

If this scenario plants seeds of paranoia in your mind, the best thing you can do is to remember that PPH is a relatively unusual event. However, if your partner does experience excessive bleeding during or after the birth, your role as her calm and confident supporter is all the more essential. Follow any instructions from the midwife, keep the birth space warm, and reassure your partner that she and her baby are safe.

Ray's Story
Suspense and joy

Ray is an information technology manager from Chicago who confesses to being a bit 'crunchy' in his outlook. The tragic death of his first wife from an asthma attack made him all too aware of life's fragility, but that experience only strengthened his conviction to welcome his first baby with his second wife, Mary, at home. Ray's faith in the normality of birth helped him to support Mary through a long labour and a postpartum haemorrhage. Fortunately for all concerned, the outcome was a positive one, and Ray's belief in home birth has only been reinforced by his experience.

From the start, Graeme impressed us with his timing. We were awaiting the arrival of some friends from Colorado, one of whom had experience attending births as a doula. They were planning to stay with us and visit some family in the area, so that they would be able to assist as long as the baby arrived during the weeks just before or after the due date. We looked forward to their visit, and anticipated having a few days after their arrival to socialise and show them around the city, but it did not turn out quite that way.
Our friends arrived late in the afternoon a week before Mary was due, and by the time we got them settled in, ate, and chatted a bit, it was time for bed. That night, at 3am, Mary awakened me to announce that she had been having contractions for two hours already. There was nothing else to do; we stayed in bed for another couple of hours, and I helped her through the contractions the best I could.

The next 18 hours were a marathon of trying to make Mary as comfortable as possible. Every few minutes, Mary winced and moaned, coping with the pain. We walked, sat, leaned, used pillows, held hands, and even spent time in the shower. We kept ice water and electrolyte beverages within arm's reach, and I brought anything else she asked for. I embraced her, massaged her, and breathed with her.

At a more decent hour that morning, we called the midwife practice to let them know that the game was afoot. Later in the afternoon, we called again to let them know that the contractions were closer together, and lasting longer. About the time the midwife and her assistant arrived, Mary tried the tub, which seemed to help her relax between contractions.

A bit later, Mary announced that she wanted me in the tub with her. She had already pooped in the water (something they don't seem to show in the water birth videos), but I didn't hesitate to strip down and climb in. Somewhere along the way, that morning and afternoon, I had become connected to Mary more deeply than I had ever experienced before. She was enduring massive pain for both of us and for the baby, and I wasn't about to let a little bit of discomfort or squeamishness on my part prevent me from assisting her in any way that I could. I held her in the water, and was extremely gratified when she was able to relax and lean against me.

Toward the evening, Mary's progress stalled. She was getting tired, and rightfully so, after all the effort she had expended. The midwife kept tabs on the baby, checking its heart rate every so often. There was no immediate cause for concern, but the longer the labour lasted, the more the risk of fetal stress increased. Mary had 'clicked' with the midwife's assistant, so the midwife decided to clear the room except for the assistant, to see if they could work together. At first I felt guilty for the break and thought I should be in there helping! But after a while, I became grateful. I hadn't realised how exhausted I was, giving Mary so much energy and attention for so many hours without eating or resting myself.

So the last few hours of labour became like a vigil for our friends and me. I don't really remember much of what we did, other than sit and talk and eat a bit. Our focus was still upstairs, of course, where the midwife went periodically to check on Mary's progress. We anxiously awaited her reports when she returned. Eventually, she went up to check, and she didn't come back down. Finally, the word was passed: if I was going to see the birth, it was time go upstairs.

When I arrived back in the room, Mary was pushing with all she had at each contraction. A few minutes later, the baby crowned. It had hair! It slipped back inside, then came a bit further out on the next push. Progress seemed agonisingly slow because of Mary's pain and effort, but I think that by this time it was actually proceeding fairly well. She tried a couple of different positions and ended up squatting against a wall. I knelt down on one side of her, with the assistant on the other. More and more of the head came out, and my excitement grew. Finally, the entire head was out, and on the next push, the baby rocketed out astonishingly fast. If my hands had been relied on to receive it, its head would have hit the floor! Fortunately, the assistant deftly caught the baby, and then there was a blur of motion as she and the midwife checked it out to make sure everything was OK, wiped it off a bit, and got it into Mary's arms on her chest as fast as possible. It breathed! But I honestly don't remember if it cried. After a moment, still not knowing the baby's sex, I blurted out, 'What is it?' We pulled the blanket aside and lifted a leg . . . it was a boy!

We were all thrilled and relieved, but the process wasn't finished yet. We transferred mother and child to the bed, and about 45 minutes later, Mary delivered the placenta. Then things became scary, as Mary kept bleeding. And bleeding. The midwife worked to stop it, without success at first. Then she asked me to take the baby downstairs to wait it out.

The next hour was one of the longest in my life, as we all waited anxiously, baby Graeme in my arms. I was worried. Having lost my first wife to an asthma attack, I was keenly aware that death can and does happen, and I didn't sign up to be a single parent right from the start. But the midwife was also an experienced RN [registered nurse], fully qualified to administer the necessary drugs, and to stitch up the tearing that had occurred. Finally, she came back downstairs, and we all breathed a sigh of relief. Mary was OK, having received treatment equal, if not superior, to what she would have received in the hospital.

What if there is a genuine emergency and we have to go to the hospital? How can I be helpful without freaking out, and how can I forgive myself if something goes wrong?

Fortunately, the vast majority of women who plan to deliver at home end up doing exactly that. The largest North American study of home births found that only 12.1% of those women who had planned home births at the onset of labour were transferred to a hospital,[13] while a similar study in the UK put the transfer rate at 16%.[14] Of those women who do go to hospital, failure to progress is widely cited as the main reason for the move, rather than any kind of immediate, catastrophic emergency. If you think that a hospital transfer has to involve the wailing sirens and screeching tires of an ambulance, you may be reassured to know that this scenario, although real, is actually quite rare.

The hospital environment may be very different from the cosy ambiance of your home, but your role as protector of the birth space remains very much the same. You may no longer be able to control the 'guest list', light your partner's favourite candles, or play her favourite music, but you can still try to ensure that she is treated with dignity and respect. Ask for medical staff to explain your partner's options whenever possible, and don't be shy in requesting a moment of private discussion time when important choices need to be made. Even if events have taken an unexpected turn, your partner can still take ownership of the birth process if she is allowed to make informed choices about her care. She may be pressured to agree to certain procedures (and you may be pressured to act as a 'voice of reason' on the doctors' behalf), but one thing remains constant in the journey from home to hospital: your partner's basic human right to give birth to her child in the manner of her choosing.

In many instances, the midwife who attended your partner at home will be able to accompany you to the labour suite, providing another welcome element of continuity. Your doula, if you have one, may be also able to offer reassurance and support. If you feel that you are at risk of 'freaking out', then don't hesitate to ask your birth team for a bit of extra back-up. The hospital environment may be unfamiliar and daunting to you but it is a familiar workplace for midwives and doulas. They can help to interpret the goings-on in the labour ward, and they can stay with your partner if you need to step outside for a quiet moment to yourself.

In the unlikely event of a genuine emergency, you may be overwhelmed by a wave of mixed emotions: gratitude for the intervention of modern medicine, but disappointment that intervention was necessary; relief because of the safe arrival of your baby, but disappointment in yourself for failing to anticipate or prevent complications. You may despair at the impersonal nature of hospital-based care, while wondering, at the same time, whether you should ever have agreed to birth at home. The answers may not come easily, but the process of asking questions is an important and healthy step towards understanding your baby's birth and moving forward into conscious parenting.

The following stories may provide some insight into two worst-case scenarios. In one, postpartum haemorrhage poses a life-threatening challenge to a mother's life; in the other, a breech twin birth prompts a frantic dash to the hospital. Both fathers share their shock and sadness as they tell their stories, but they also share their lasting conviction that home was the best place for their children to be born. Perhaps not all fathers would feel the same; these stories address deeply personal issues which you and your partner might wish to discuss after reading these heartfelt accounts.

Willie's story
A close call

Willie, a car dealer from just outside Glasgow, Scotland, initially found it difficult to accept his wife's desire for a home birth. His two children from a previous marriage and his first child with Debbie had all been born by emergency Caesarean section, and Willie had learned to associate birth with trauma. However, Debbie soon persuaded him, and she went on to have a triumphant home water birth. Unfortunately, a catastrophic bleed after the birth required a stay in the hospital but, as Willie explains below, that experience has only deepened his appreciation of the intimacy of home birth.

Debbie started getting twinges in the early hours of the morning, and she began wondering whether this was the start of labour. As it progressed, the pain became a lot more painful than she'd probably thought it would be in the initial stages. That's when the TENS machine came on, and then Debbie phoned the doula at about 5.30am.

Debbie was trying to keep herself busy with a few things, doing things around the house and getting prepared, and I was just following her and asking what she wanted me to do – menial tasks like making something to eat, making some tea, or tidying up. One of my big jobs was looking after the water in the birth pool. Because I didn't know when Debbie was going to get into it, I was concerned whether I had enough hot water to keep it at a constant temperature, and wondering if it was going to fall through the floorboards!

When the doula came, Debbie calmed down a bit because she had somebody there to support her and to understand how she was feeling, so I tended to just watch from that point on, and anything that had to be done, I would do it. Obviously I was looking at Debbie and giving her a wee cuddle now and again to reassure her that I was supporting her, but I was unable to do anything else in that sense. You do feel a little bit lost, as if, 'What should I be doing?' You walk around in circles a bit as a man, but it's just a case of being there.

I also had to try and make arrangements to get our son housed somewhere else for the big event, because he would have been distressed seeing and hearing his mum in pain – one thing I wasn't prepared for was the noise that a pregnant woman can make! So I got him dressed, fed, and watered, and made arrangements to have him taken away.

Debbie was trying to find comfortable positions throughout the house. She would lie on the couch, the floor, the bed; she'd be down on all fours. I can remember her face almost like she'd run a marathon, and there was a lot of pain and tiredness in her eyes, and I was wondering how much longer she could carry on like that. You could see her energy levels draining away. She and the doula decided to call the midwives, and they arrived soon after that.

Debbie laboured on for a while, but then the midwives made a decision to call an ambulance. I think there was a problem; they weren't exactly sure if the baby was moving down the birth canal quick enough or whether it was in distress. They also felt Debbie was getting extremely tired, and maybe they thought she couldn't cope any further. I was worried that the ambulance wouldn't be able to find the house, so I went outside and waited down at the end of the drive to help them find us – that also gave me something to do, menial as it was at the time.

The ambulance came 20 minutes later and I guided it up the road, but by then, the midwives had decided that they actually didn't need it, so I had to go and tell the paramedics to go away. It was a gamble for the midwives – the ambulance would have had a bit more equip.m.ent than they would have had in the house, and the transfer time from the house to the hospital would have been 25 to 30 minutes, but I was confident in the midwives and I think they knew that the birth was imminent.

After I came back in the house, I could still see some fear in the midwives' faces, but then, after Debbie made a few comments demanding a transfer to the hospital and a C-section, I remember them looking at each other in a quietly confident way, as if to say, 'The baby's coming now!' My task then was to hold the torch onto the water, and that to me was probably the most vivid memory of the whole birth: seeing the baby's head appearing through the torchlight and then slipping out and coming up to the surface. That's an experience I'll never, ever forget.

Once Jessica was born, there was a calm. The love surrounding the home was fantastic. I could see the happiness in Debbie's face, that she had managed to do this, and I was immensely proud of her for doing it. The midwives and the doula left and we were a little family unit; it was blissful, it was lovely. That lasted for a couple of hours. Debbie had a shower, got dressed, and fed the baby. Then she said she was starting to get some pain, almost like labour pain, and it didn't go away; it started getting worse and worse. She knew it wasn't right so she phoned the labour ward; they told her it was just the womb contracting, but she came off the phone and said that something was definitely wrong. She phoned again, and then she just started fading. She was bleeding and it was as if the life was just bleeding out of her. I spoke to the labour ward and told them that we needed an ambulance; that Debbie was bleeding and it wasn't stopping or clotting.

Debbie was sitting on one couch, the baby was on the other couch, I was in between, and there was a period of about twenty minutes where I felt as if there was absolutely nothing I could do. I thought Debbie was going to die; she was just sitting there. She managed to nod when I spoke to her but she couldn't speak to me. I tried to contain the bleeding as much as possible, and I phoned the ambulance again to make sure it was on its way.

Eventually, the ambulance came, and two paramedics came in. They took Debbie out to the ambulance on a stretcher and kept her there for about twenty minutes. I later learned that they were giving her some IV treatment to get her fluids back up, and if they hadn't done that, she wouldn't have made it to the hospital.

I asked the paramedics what to do about the baby – she was still only two hours old, but she'd been fed and was quite content. They told me that I would need to bring her into the hospital, so after Debbie went away in the ambulance, I had to phone a friend to come round and help me find some baby clothes and things. We got the baby seat out and got the baby into the car; it was a freezing cold night. I drove up to the hospital with this two-hour-old baby, not knowing what state my wife would be in.

When I got to the hospital, it was very much like you see on the TV programmes; I got taken into a little side room, and these two young doctors came in and said they'd do what they could for Debbie – not what I wanted to hear. They said they could take the baby and look after her, so I then went into the room where Debbie was and there was a medical team of maybe six or eight people there. Debbie was conscious, she'd come round, and they were waiting for the consultant to come and for the units of blood to arrive.

When the consultant finally came, to be honest, his attitude was very bolshy. He said, 'What's happened here? A home birth?', and I could see that he thought, 'Why have I been called out to something like this? This shouldn't have happened; this woman should have been in the hospital.' Although Debbie was in pain, she fought with him and gave her opinion on that, and i think he was a bit shocked and taken aback!

In hindsight, we know that the PPH could have happened in the hospital, it could have happened anywhere. They never gave us a specific reason why it occurred; I certainly remember the midwives at home looking at the placenta and saying that it was perfect, and that everything had come away. Debbie said to me that if she'd been in hospital, she could have been tucked up in bed, the midwives could have left her to sleep, and they might never have discovered the bleeding, so the outcome could have actually been a lot worse in the hospital! But the PPH was certainly not due to the home birth at all. Not at all.

Absolutely without a doubt, I still feel like we did the right thing having a home birth. Would I do it again? That's a big question. Knowing what I know now, if we were going to have another child, I probably would support Debbie in having a home birth again. My knowledge of it is a bit deeper now. You still have fears whether you're in the hospital or not, but the closeness and the involvement I had was 100 times better at home than it would have been in the hospital. Yes, I would support her.

James' Story
Making decisions and sticking with them

James and his wife, Gail, are both nurses in the south of England. Gail's pregnancy with twins raised eyebrows from the outset, but with a bit of persistence and the support of her local midwifery team, Gail was able to realise her dream of birthing both babies at home. The difficult delivery and subsequent hospitalisation of the second twin have made James and Gail question their birth choices on a fundamental level, but the challenges their family has faced have only strengthened their resolve.

It all started when our first daughter, Eve, who's now two, was born at home. We had a very positive experience, it was a completely safe pregnancy with no complications, and there were no institutional obstacles to having Eve at home. What appealed to me about home birth was the fact that you're in your natural environment, you feel relaxed and comfortable. You feel more in control because it's your place, it's on your terms, and it also doesn't involved any disruption, having to go to another place or travel or that kind of thing. So when Gail became pregnant again, we wanted the same thing. We found out during our scan that there were twins, but we wanted to continue with having them at home.

There are a lot of obstacles to being able to have a choice to have twins at home. I think there has only been one other twin home birth on the NHS in this wider area that we're in. It just doesn't happen, midwives don't have experience delivering twins at home, and it is not recommended. Twin pregnancies are seen as being a lot more risky than singletons, and that message is spelled out to you quite clearly from the start; really, under no circumstances would you be advised to even consider a home birth. The odds were very much stacked against us.

Also, we wanted to have midwifery-led care. We feel that consultant-led care takes a bit of control away from you and medicalises birth unnecessarily. We didn't even see a doctor when we had Eve because there was never any need to. With the twin pregnancy, we had to see the consultant on one occasion antenatally. The staff were very nice but they made it very clear that what we were doing had to be written in capital letters in the notes – 'You're doing this against the medical profession's advice!' We felt like the consultant put far too much focus on risk. There wasn't much focus on what the positives were of being at home, and what the positives were of having a normal twin pregnancy.

In our local community, midwifery services are excellent. The midwives are quite a stable, cohesive team of people. We had excellent midwifery care with Eve, and to be completely honest, we've had excellent care this time around as well. From early on, we were very persistent with wanting to have a home birth, if it was possible. We never said, 'We want a home birth no matter what, and we're not going to listen to what anyone else says.' It wasn't like that. If Gail had a healthy pregnancy, and everything went smoothly, and there weren't any obvious risks, then this was something we wanted to do. Once people became aware that we were actually serious about it, and that we wouldn't change our minds, it was a question of enlisting the support of the community midwives. In order to do that, part of the care had to be shared with the senior members of the team who were willing to support our choice. Some of the midwives in the team weren't willing to be on our rota, partly because they hadn't had the experience of delivering twins at home.

The pregnancy went really well, although there was one complication. The second twin was initially head down, but it turned breech during the pregnancy, which presented a potential obstacle, but we were still supported in being able to have them at home. The pregnancy went just over full term,

a couple of days past 40 weeks. We were starting to get a bit concerned because you have to get to 37 weeks to have a home birth here, and then once we did, we were willing things to happen. Gail then started wondering how long she would be allowed to go until she had to be induced.
Gail went into labour spontaneously at about five o'clock in the morning, in the midst of quite a hot spell that we'd been having. She laboured well. I had a fairly active role in supporting her, emotionally and practically – I made the calls to the midwife, got things organised in the house, and sent our daughter out with Gail's mum, who'd been staying with us. We had a birth plan and I helped Gail to go through that. Also, Gail didn't have any pain relief during the labour – she had wanted gas and air, but decided not to – so I was helping her to manage her breathing and keeping her mentally focused.

There were three midwives in attendance for the actual births. The first twin was born just about quarter past midday: a boy, Jack. He came head-first in the normal position. Gail was on all fours and I was at her head. It was incredibly intense. I was calm, but it was difficult to keep my emotions under control – there were some tears! And the funny thing with twins is that once the first one's out, you've got that incredibly joyous release of emotion, and then it's like, oh my goodness, we've got to do the same thing again! And of course we knew the second child was breech, which could potentially be problematic.

Gail was squatting by this time, and our daughter Cara's legs came out first, but it took time for the rest of the body and the head to be delivered, and Gail's contractions had slowed down a bit, so she changed position and lay on her back. We then realised that the cord was around Cara's neck, and she was blue when she came out. Then it became quite traumatic. The midwives whipped Cara off next door to massage her heart and to ventilate her. Gail and I were in shock. I won't go into the detail of what happened, but we had to call an ambulance straight away, and I had to go with Cara and one of the midwives in the ambulance. Gail stayed at home with one of the midwives and Jack. I was in pieces. Our worst nightmare had happened.

It was extremely revealing being in hospital for that time, afterwards, because it's very hard to feel like you're in control in a hospital environment. The service was excellent, I can't fault anyone, but it's quite harsh, and very medicalised.

Cara had to spend a bit of time in special care, but three weeks on, she's actually doing really well. She's growing, she's feeding, and she's fine. There are one or two things we won't know about her until she develops, because of the trauma, but our fingers are crossed that there won't be any permanent damage. Fortunately, things have worked out well for Cara.

In terms of home birth, we've had to ask ourselves a lot of questions about it and do some soul searching. Was it the right thing to do? Would things have been different if the twins had been born in hospital? On balance, to be completely honest, we wouldn't have done a thing differently. Primarily, you can't live your life thinking about what could have been and what might have been – you've got to make decisions and stick with them. Also, if we had laboured in hospital, Cara still would have been born the same way, and she would have had the same trauma. OK, she would have been closer to the 'crash team' [emergency team] and that kind of thing, but the midwives at home did that part of the work very, very well. They massaged her and got her going straight away – there wasn't a delay where she was out for any length of time, they got her ventilated straight away, the ambulance was here very quickly, we got to hospital very quickly. So there was trauma, but we'd do the same thing tomorrow. It was an amazing experience, and being at home was one of the most amazing things about it.

7

Now what?

It's four o'clock in the morning and your home looks as if it's been hit by some kind of New Age hurricane. Half-empty bottles of essential oils lie strewn across the living room floor, and the smell of jasmine and clary sage mingle with the breeze from an open window. A couple of candles are burning low in the corner. On tables and shelves around the room, other candles have melted into soft, waxy puddles. Towels, pillows and your partner's bathrobe snake a messy trail towards the bedroom, where the woman you love has drifted into the deepest sleep of her life, your newborn baby curled in the crook of her arm. Your home is a mess. Your home, you think, has never looked better.

Many of the fathers who contributed to this book were deeply moved by the feelings of euphoria and calm that followed their home births. In the comments below, they describe a kind of postnatal 'bubble' around their homes and their families:

> *There was a lot of physical and emotional energy through the birth, and so for a few hours afterwards, I felt that still lingered in the house. It was a fantastic feeling, just the three of us being left on our own to enjoy the moment. That lasted for a few days, that happiness. I was over the moon about the birth process and having a cute baby boy. For Sophie, it was much more deep and profound, but I basked in that feeling around her. (Chi)*

The first few days were just euphoric – we just could not believe that we had managed to produce this beautiful little boy. (David N.)

It was just like the first three days after our wedding. We were just 'floating'. (Jorge)

There are any number of reasons why parents might experience these feelings of deep contentment after a home birth gone right: delight with the new baby, triumph at having achieved their birth goals (sometimes in the face of substantial opposition), and mutual appreciation of each other's efforts during the birth itself.

Because their baby was born at home, both parents can weave the birth seamlessly into the fabric of their normal family life. In the hospital, a man may be allowed a 'grace period' of a few hours to enjoy his new baby before he is hustled away from a busy ward, and in the days that follow, the process of admiring and supporting this new life is punctuated by trips to the hospital canteen, frustrated fumblings with the baby's new car seat, and efforts to feed hungry parking meters. Home-birthing fathers, by contrast, enjoy a sense of continuity in the early postnatal period:

Because we'd had the birth at home, it just flowed into family life. It wasn't like we were 'Coming Home'; we were already here, and we seamlessly just went straight into it. (Bob)

There were no car seats to strap the baby into. Instead of welcoming the baby into the home, we brought her outside to welcome her to the neighbourhood ... It almost felt as if, not only had we accomplished something, but also that the community itself had helped bring this baby into the world. (Geoff)

These 'modern' men are echoing the experiences of generations of families in indigenous cultures around the world, for whom birth is not an isolated event shared by two parents and a team of highly skilled strangers in a hospital. Rather, birth is viewed as an event that is both mundane and extraordinary, one that is celebrated by the community but also accepted as a normal part of family life.

You might also look to the wisdom of indigenous cultures as you try to organise your postnatal home at a practical level. A quick look at modern Western tabloids would have you believe that the days after a birth are spent sterilising bottles and making trips to the gym to get rid of the infamous 'mummy tummy'. In reality, the hours, days and weeks that follow any birth, anywhere, are a crucial window of time during which the family's new dynamic is created, for better or for worse. Many indigenous cultures have a traditional 'lying-in' time of 20 to 40 days after a birth, when the new mother rests, bonds with her baby, and is attended by female friends and relatives. Sometimes, the father contributes to this special time by praying for the health of his new family, by keeping a fire burning to warm his wife's space, or by preparing special foods to nourish and delight her. Although we have no similar rituals in the industrialised West, the desire for peaceful intimacy in the days after a birth is universal and can be easily satisfied after a home birth. You can continue your role as protector of the birth space by limiting the number of non-essential visitors to the home, relieving your partner of housework for a while, and keeping any older siblings occupied. As one father noted, 'A rested wife is a blessed life.'

What if I don't feel so joyful or blessed after the birth? Do other men feel like that, too?

While a normal birth at home is usually a happy event for all concerned, any birth also brings major changes to the family dynamic. In the short term, your partner must focus almost all of her physical and emotional energy on the baby, and what little energy is left must be used for preserving her own wellbeing with the odd hour of sleep and some high-calorie eating. If your partner is breastfeeding, then she will be in the process of giving her body over to this new life in a way that is intimate and complete. This process can be amazing to watch, but it can also raise feelings of insecurity, envy and loss in even the most supportive man. You might wonder whether, in the long term, your partner will ever have the time and energy to include you in her attentions.

This period can be all the more challenging if your home birth has not gone according to plan. If your partner ended up having more interventions than she had wanted and/or if she required transfer to a hospital, then you may still be reeling from this unanticipated and unwelcome turn of events. It is completely normal to experience feelings of guilt, anger and remorse under these circumstances: you might find it difficult to stop replaying the birth in your head, wondering whether you should have made different choices or how you might have 'saved' the situation with a cooler head or a quicker reaction. Of course, nobody can control a birth, and its elemental unpredictably is what makes it so awe-inspiring. However, this may be of little consolation if you are grieving the loss of the perfect home birth that might have been, but never was.

Regardless of whether your baby's birth was triumphantly straightforward or disappointingly complex, it may be helpful to talk about the experience, first with your partner but then, also, with somebody who is slightly removed from the situation. Acknowledge the power of the birth experience; take pleasure in what was joyful and reflect on what was not. Telling and re-telling your birth story may help to put the event into perspective, and you may find it reassuring to go over what happened, when, and why. This kind of debriefing may be difficult in a world where men are hardly encouraged to share their feelings openly, but it is interesting to note that in the absence of face-to-face camaraderie, many new fathers are finding a new forum for their thoughts, namely, online weblogs, or 'blogs'. Here, one man describes how writing a blog allowed him to share his feelings about home birth and parenthood more freely than his usual social circle might permit:

> *I put the birth online on the blog, because it felt like I could share it. At times, I felt it was difficult [to debrief]; female friends will listen to the birth story in its full length and male friends will listen to the story in a much more abbreviated version and then say, 'Anyway, let's have a pint,' and then they'll move on quite swiftly to talk about something else. It's not that you want to bore people, but you do kind of want to go, 'I've got my baby and that's all I do now, and I'm quite happy with that,' and it's difficult to convey that to other people who haven't got that, and who aren't very interested, to be honest. (Bob)*

Finding a safe, non-judgmental audience for your thoughts about the birth – whether it be online or face to face – can be a valuable way of processing your experience and reaffirming your values as you move forward into parenthood.

How can I carry the lessons I've learned from my home birth with me into the rest of my life as a father?

It's not surprising that witnessing a home birth in all of its challenging, unhindered glory gives many men a newfound respect and appreciation for their partners:

> *I didn't have a negative perception of my wife beforehand. However, I have a very limited imagination, and that handicaps my sense of what she is capable of. The home births showed me how the problem didn't lie with her perceived shortcomings, but rather with my own inability to trust her instincts. (Geoff)*

> *I can't even imagine what she went through, but my admiration level went through the roof. She did an amazing job for our children and family! I love her so much more!!!!! (Jorge)*

What may be even more surprising is the newfound respect many men have for *themselves* after supporting their partners through birth at home. The men who contributed to this book spoke with pride about their roles as fathers, protectors and birth partners:

> *The birth gave me more confidence in life . . . You feel like you can look after your family, you feel more equipped to do that. (Murray)*
>
> *I think I am more likely to take a risk now than I was before. I am probably more sceptical of the 'official line,' especially when it comes to the medical establishment. I feel like I am capable of taking on more responsibility for my own choices than I was before. (Geoff)*
>
> *I never thought that I would be so involved and play such an important role for my wife. It changed all of our lives completely. (Jorge)*
>
> *The births were the highlights of my life. They helped me feel better about myself as a man and as a father. (David S)*

You, too, will be transformed by the birth of your child, no matter where it occurs. Birth takes its participants to a place they have never been before, but it is only one leg of the longer journey that is parenthood. In thinking about home birth, you and your partner have already begun to work together to make the best choices for your family. Take that wisdom with you on the rest of your journey – and enjoy it.

Epilogue

So you've finished the book, and maybe in the course of reading it, you and your partner have had a baby. How was it for you? Have you become a home birth evangelist, or does the thought of birth without doctors bring you out in a rash? Either way, go out and *talk about it.* Tell a friend, a colleague, a cousin, a brother. Tell your own father, if you can. As Geoff from Pennsylvania puts it:

> ***Be sure to share your story. There is no shortage of fear-mongering and simply unhelpful advice when it comes to birth. As fathers, we need to make birth a part of the masculine dialogue.***

References

1 Risk and Responsibility

1 Department of Health. Changing Childbirth: Report of the Expert Maternity Group Part 1. London: HMSO, 1993.

2 Tew M. Do obstetric intranatal interventions make birth safer? British Journal of Obstetric Gynaecology 1986; 93: 659-674.

3 Northern Regional Perinatal Mortality Survey Coordinating Group. Collaborative survey of perinatal loss in planned and unplanned home births. British Medical Journal 1996; 313: 1306-1309.

4 Ackermann-Liebrich U, Voegeli T, Gunter-Witt K, Kunzi I, Zullig M, Schindler C, Maurer M, and Zurich Study Team. Home versus hospital deliveries: follow up study of matched pairs for procedures and outcome. British Medical Journal 1996; 313: 1313-1318.

5 Wiegers TA, Keirse MJNC, van der Zee J, and Berghs GAH. Outcome of planned home and planned hospital births in low risk pregnancies: prospective study in midwifery practices in the Netherlands. British Medical Journal 1996; 313: 1309-1313.

6 Olsen O. Meta.analysis of the safety of home births. Birth 1997; 24(1): 4-13.

7 Chamberlain G, Wraight A, and Crowley P. Home Births: The Report of the 1994 Confidential Enquiry by the National Birthday Trust Fund. New York and London: Parthenon, 1997.

8 Young G, Hey E. Home birth in Britain can be safe. British Medical Journal 2000; 320: 798.

9 Johnson KC, Daviss B. Outcomes of planned home births with certified professional midwives: large prospective study in North America. British Medical Journal 2005; 330: 1416.

10 Royal College of Obstetricians and Gynaecologists and Royal College of Midwives. Joint Statement No. 2, April 2007. www.rcog.org.uk/index.asp?PageID=2023 (accessed 13 September 2008).

11 Department of Health. National service framework for children, young people, and maternity services: Executive summary. London: HMSO, 1994.

12 Department of Health. Maternity matters: choice, access, and continuity of care in a safe service. London: HMSO, 1997.

13 American College of Obstetricians and Gynecologists Statement on Home Births, February 6, 2008. www.acog.org/from_home/publications/press_releases/nr02-06-08-2.cfm (accessed 13 September, 2008).

14 Hunter, A. Are Home Births Dangerous? ABC News online. July 11 2008. www.abcnews.go.com/Health/Story?id=5340949&page=2 (accessed 11 September 2008).

15 Enkin M, Keirse MJNC, Chalmers I. A Guide to Effective Care in Pregnancy and Childbirth: Third Edition. Oxford: Oxford University Press, 2000.

16 Central Intelligence Agency. The World Factbook: Infant mortality rates. www.cia.gov (accessed 2 September 2008).

17 Save The Children. 2007 Mother's Index. www.savethechildren.org/campaigns/state-of-the-worlds-mothers-report/2007/mothers-index.html (accessed 13 September 2008).

18 Wagner M. Fish can't see water: the need to humanize birth. International Journal of Gynecology and Obstetrics 2001; 75: supplement s25-37.

19 Yance MK, Clark P, Duff P. The frequency of glove contamination during cesarean delivery. Obstetric Gynaecology 1994 April; 83(4): 538–542.

20 Chapman S, Duff P. Frequency of blood perforations and subsequent blood contact in association with selected obstetric surgical procedures. American Journal of Obstetrics and Gynecology 1993 May; 168(5): 1354-7.

21 Health Protection Agency / Communicable Disease Surveillance Centre. Surveillance of surgical site infection in English hospitals 1997-2002. www.hpa.org.uk (accessed 2 September 2008).

22 Association for Professionals in Infection Control & Epidemiology. National prevalence study of methicillin-resistant staphylococcus aureus (MRSA) in US healthcare facilities. www.apic.org/content/navigationmenu/researchfoundation/previousstudies/nationalmrsaprevalencestudy/apic_mrsa_study_exec.pdf (accessed 2 September 2008).

23 Thomas, P. Your Birth Rights. London: The Women's Press, 2002.

24 Downe S, McCormick S, Beech B. Labour interventions associated with normal birth. British Journal of Midwifery, 9 (10): 602-606.

25 Beech, B. Am I Allowed? Surbiton, Surrey: Association for Improvements in the Maternity Services, 2003.

26 Edwards NP. Birthing Autonomy: Women's Experiences of Planning Home Births. London: Routledge, 2005.

27 Biesele M. An ideal of unassisted birth: hunting, healing, and transformation. In Davis-Floyd R, Sargent CF (eds.). Childbirth and authoritative knowledge: cross-cultural perspectives. Berkeley, CA: University of California Press, 1997.

28 Wesson N. Home Birth: A Practical Guide. London: Pinter and Martin, 2006.

29 Kitzinger S. Homebirth. London: Dorling Kindersley, 1991.

30 Vause S., Macintosh M. Use of prostaglandins to induce labour in women with a Caesarean section scar. British Medical Journal 1999; 318: 1056-1058.

31 Miller DA, Diaz, FG, Paul RH. Vaginal birth after Caesarean: a 10-year experience. Obstetric Gynaecology 1994 Aug; 84: 255-258.

32 Chippington-Derrick D. Aftershock. AIMS Journal 2007; 19(1): 8.

33 Various contributors. Breech presentation: options for care. In Informed choice for professionals. Bristol: MIDIRS, 2005.

34 Cronk M. Keep your hands off the breech. AIMS Journal 2005, 17(1). www.aims.org.uk/Journal/Vol10No3/handOffbreech.htm (accessed 14 September 2008).

35 Edwards *op cit.*

36 Furin K. Personal conversation on 6 February 2008.

37 Odent M. Birth Reborn. London: Souvenir Press, 1984.

38 Ford C, Iliffe S, and Owen F. Outcome of planned homebirths in an inner city practice. British Medical Journal 1991; 303 (6816): 1517-1519.

39 Demilew J. Southeast London midwifery group practice. MIDIRS Midwifery Journal 1994, 4(3): 270-272.

40 Furin *op cit.*

2 Think Positive

1 Arlen H, Mercer J. 'Ac-cent-tchu-ate the positive,' for Here Come The Waves, Paramount Pictures, 1944.

2 Mander R. Men and Maternity. London: Routledge, 2004.

3 Milne F. Fathering from within. Juno 2008; 14: 31.

3 Choosing the Guest List

1 Odent *op cit.*

2 Midwifery Task Force, Inc. The Midwives Model of Care. www.cfmidwifery.org/mmoc/define.aspx (accessed 5 September 2008).

3 Gaskin IM. Spiritual Midwifery. Summertown, Tennessee: Book Publishing Company, 2002.

4 Klaus MH., Kennell JH, Klaus PH. Mothering the Mother: How a Doula Can Help You Have a Shorter, Easier, and Healthier Birth. New York: Addison-Wesley Publishing Company, 1993.

5 Kitzinger, Homebirth, *op cit.*

6 Thomas *op cit.*

7 Gaskin IM. Some thoughts on unassisted childbirth. Midwifery Today, 2003 Summer: 38-40.

8 Burnett CA 3rd, Jones JA, Rooks J, Chen CH, Tyler CW Jr, Miller CA. Home delivery and neonatal mortality in North Carolina. Journal of the American Medical Association 1980 Dec 19; 244(24): 2741–2745.

9 Haloob R, Thein A. Born before arrival, a five year retrospective controlled study. Journal of Obstetrics and Gynaecology 1992 Mar; 12(2): 100-104.

10 Murphy JF, Dauncey M, Gray OP, Chalmers I. Planned and unplanned deliveries at home: implications of a changing ratio. British Medical Journal 1984 May 12; 288(6428): 1429-1432.

11 Giving birth without a midwife or doctor. www.aims.org.uk/homebirthUpdated.htm (accessed 5 September 2008).

12 Beech *op cit.*

4 Pleasure and Pain

1 Houser, P. Fathers-To-Be Handbook. Lamberhurst, Kent: Creative Life Systems Ltd, 2007.

2 Balaskas J. New Active Birth. London: Thorsons, 1989.

3 Kitzinger, Rediscovering Birth. London: Little, Brown, 2000.

4 Odent M. Primal Health. East Sussex: Clairview, 2002.

5 Smith, CA, Collins, CT, Cyna, AM, Crowther, CA. Complementary and alternative therapies for pain management in labour. Cochrane Database Systematic Review, 2003; (2): CD003521.

6 Burns E, Blamey C. Complementary medicine. Using aromatherapy in childbirth. Nursing Times, 1994 Mar 2-8; 90(9): 54-60.

7 Balaskas J. The Water Birth Book. London: Thorsons, 2004

8 Sky News, see www.news.sky.com/skynews/Home/Sky-News-Archive/Article/20082851285755?f=rss (accessed 5 September 2008).

9 Stockton, A. Positive Pain. Self-published, 2006.

10 Calvert J, Steen M. Homepathic remedies for self-administration during childbirth. British Journal of Midwifery 2007 Mar; 15(3): 159-165.

11 Various contributors. Non-epidural strategies for pain relief during labour. In Informed Choice for Professionals. Bristol: MIDIRS, 2005.

5 Birth: Normal and Extraordinary

1 Yildrim G, Beji NK. Effects of pushing techniques in birth on mother and fetus: a randomized study. Birth 2008 Mar; 35(1): 25-30(6).

2 Hutton E, Hassan ES. Late versus early clamping of the umbilical cord in full-term neonates: systematic review and meta-analysis of controlled trials. Journal of the American Medical Association 2007; 297(11): 1241-52.

3 BBC News online. www.news.bbc.co.uk/2/hi/uk_news/magazine/4918290.stm (accessed 5 September 2008).

6 Challenges and Complications

1 Olsen SJ, Secher NJ. Low consumption of seafood in early pregnancy as a risk factor for preterm delivery: prospective cohort study. British Medical Journal 2002; 324: 447.

2 Dooley MM, Studd J. Prolonged pregnancy. In Turnbull A, Chamberlain G (eds.). Obstetrics. Edinburgh: Churchill Livingstone, 1989: 771-81.

3 Papiernik E, Alexander GR, and Paneth N. Racial differences in pregnancy duration and its implications for perinatal care. Medical Hypotheses 1990; 33(3): 181-6.

4 Zhu JL, Hjollund NH, Olsen J. Shift work, duration of pregnancy and birth weight: The National Birth Cohort in Denmark. American Journal of Obstetrics and Gynecology 2004; 191(1): 285-91.

5 Enkin et al, *op cit.*

6 US Food and Drug Administration notes on Cytotec www.fda.gov/Cder/foi/

label/2002/19268slr037.pdf (accessed 17 September 2008).

7 Plaut MM, Schwartz ML, Lubarsky SL. Uterine rupture associated with the use of misoprostol in the gravid patient with a previous cesarean section. American Journal of Obstetrics and Gynecology 1999 Jun; 180 (6 Pt 1): 1535-42.

8 Edozien LC. What do maternity statistics tell us about induction of labour? Journal of Obstetrics and Gynaecology 1999; 19(4): 343-4.

9 Berry, J. Allowed a homebirth? AIMS Journal, 18(1): 20.

10. Gaskin in Midwifery Today, *op cit.*

11 Moore ER, Anderson GC, Bergman N. Early skin-to-skin contact for mothers and their healthy newborn infants. Cochrane Database of Systematic Reviews 2007, Issue 2. Art. No.: CD003519. DOI: 10.1002/14651858.CD003519.pub2.

12 Beckmann MM, Garrett AJ. Antenatal perineal massage for reducing perineal trauma. Cochrane Database of Systematic Reviews 2006, Issue 1. Art. No.: CD005123. DOI: 10.1002/14651858.CD005123.pub2.

13 Johnson and Daviss *op cit.*

14 Wraight and Crowley *op cit.*

Index

About the author

Leah Hazard grew up in the United States and graduated from Harvard University before moving to the United Kingdom to pursue a career in journalism and the arts. The birth of her first daughter in 2003 inspired Leah to retrain as a doula, providing birth support to families in homes and hospitals across Central Scotland. In 2006, Leah experienced the joyful birth of her second daughter at home. She lives in Glasgow with her family and continues to work for positive change in the maternity services.

Notes